Community-Based Programs and Policies

This collection is focused on the provision of community-based programs and activities in health and related long-term care services that have contributed, or may in the future contribute, to social policy development.

Several of the articles in this collection deal with community-based health and long-term care program and policy initiatives that have been facilitated through federal programs such as Medicare, Medicaid and the Older Americans Act. The implementation of some of these community-based programs have significantly influenced social policy thinking regarding the beneficial effects of integrating medical and social aspects of health and long-term care services, as well as the health care team approach to the delivery of health and long-term care services. Another dimension addressed is the impact of interest groups, such as family caregivers, in advancing social policy that supports the efforts of community-based family caregivers in providing services to patients in need.

The underlying theme is how such local community programs have contributed in a variety of ways to the development of social policies at the community level that in many ways focus on the integration of health and related long-term care services and a health care team approach to the provision of such services.

The book will be of interest to community development courses in Schools of Social Work and other health professions such as Nursing and Public Health. It will also be of interest to health policy programs in public administration and other social sciences.

This book was published as a special issue of *Social Work in Public Health*.

Dr. Howard A. Palley is Professor of Social Policy and Distinguished Fellow, Institute for Human Services Policy at the School of Social Work, University of Maryland, Baltimore, Maryland, USA.

D0218048

Community-Based Programs and Policies

Contributions to social policy development in health care and health care-related services

Edited by Howard A. Palley

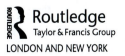

Routledge
Taylor & Francis Group

LONDON AND NEW YORK

First published 2009 by Routledge
2 Park Square, Milton Park, Abingdon, Oxon, OX14 4RN

Simultaneously published in the USA and Canada
by Routledge
270 Madison Avenue, New York, NY 10016

Routledge is an imprint of the Taylor & Francis Group, an informa business

Typeset in Times by Value Chain, India
Printed and bound in the United States of America on acid-free paper by IBT Global.

British Library Cataloguing in Publication Data
A catalogue record for this book is available from the British Library

ISBN10: 0-7890-3832-3 (HB)
ISBN10: 0-7890-3833-1 (PB)

ISBN13: 978-0-7890-3832-6 (HB)
ISBN13: 978-0-7890-3833-3 (PB)

CONTENTS

List of contributors   vii

1   Introduction   1
       Howard A. Palley

2   PACE: Has It Changed the Chronic Care Paradigm?   3
       Marty Lynch
       Mauro Hernandez
       Carroll Estes

3   Integrated Care: Incentives, Approaches,
       and Future Considerations   25
       L. Gail Dobell
       Robert J. Newcomer

4   When the Private Sphere Goes Public: Exploring
       the Issues Facing Family Caregiver Organizations
       in the Development of Long-Term Care Policies   47
       Philip A. Rozario
       Elizabeth Palley

5   Examining Fiscal Federalism, Regionalization
       and Community-Based Initiatives
       in Canada's Health Care Delivery System   67
       Pierre-Gerlier Forest
       Howard A. Palley

6   CLSCs in Quebec: Thirty Years of Community Action   87
       Benoît Gaumer
       Marie-Josée Fleury

7   Feminist Health Care in a Hostile Environment: A Case Study
      of the Womancare Health Center   105
        Cheryl A. Hyde

8   The Voice of Advocates in Health Care Policymaking
      for the Poor   123
        Colleen M. Grogan
        Michael K. Gusmano

    Index   153

LIST OF CONTRIBUTORS

L. Gail Dobell, PhD, is affiliated with the Department of Social & Behavioral Sciences, University of California, San Francisco, California.

Carroll L. Estes, PhD, is Professor, Department of Social and Behavioral Sciences, University of California, San Francisco, California.

Marie-Josée Fleury, PhD, is Associate Professor at the Department of Psychiatry, McGill University, Douglas Hospital Research Center, Verdun, Quebec.

Pierre-Gerlier Forest, PhD, is President, The Pierre Elliott Trudeau Foundation, and Associate Professor, Department of Health Administration, University of Montreal, Montreal Quebec.

Benoît Gaumer, MD, PhD, is Adjunct Professor at the Department of Health Administration, University of Montreal, Montreal Quebec.

Colleen M. Grogan, PhD, is Associate Professor at the School of Social Service Administration, University of Chicago.

Michael K. Gusmano, PhD, is Assistant Professor of Health Policy and Management, and Lauterstein Scholar at the Department of Health Policy and Management, Columbia University New York, New York.

Mauro Hernandez, PhD, is CEO of Concepts in Community Living, Inc., Clackamas, Oregon.

Cheryl A. Hyde, PhD, MSW, is Assistant Dean for Field and Continuing Education at the School of Social Administration, Temple University, Philadelphia, Pennsylvania.

Marty Lynch, PhD, is CEO, LifeLong Medical Center, Berkeley, California.

Robert J. Newcomer, PhD, is Professor at the Department of Social & Behavioral Sciences, University of California, San Francisco California.

Howard A. Palley, PhD, is Professor of Social Policy and Distinguished Fellow, Institute for Human Services Policy at the School of Social Work, University of Maryland, Baltimore, Maryland.

Philip A. Rozario, PhD, MSW and **Elizabeth Palley, PhD, JD**, are Associate Professors at the Adelphi University School of Social Work, Garden City, New York.

Introduction

Howard A. Palley

This collection is focused on community-based programs and activities that have or may in the future contribute to social policy development.

Three of our articles deal with community-based long-term care programs and policies that have been facilitated by federal financing through programs such as, Medicare, Medicaid and the Older Americans Act. In an initial article by Marty Lynch, Mauro Hernandez and Carroll Estes, the authors describe how the Program for All-Inclusive Care for the Elderly (PACE) has significantly influenced social policy thinking regarding the integration of the medical and social aspects of long-term care services. They also view PACE as having provided an influential model for breaking down the vertical silos that often have affected medical and long-term care policies and programs. A companion article by L. Gail Dobell and Robert J. Newcomer examine the various research and demonstration programs sponsored by the U.S. Centers for Medicare and Medicaid Services and discuss several programs delivered in local communities such as Disease Management and PACE and the contributions of such programs to case integration and social policy development. Their article especially emphasizes the collaborative efforts of health and social services professionals that occur within the PACE program. A third article by Philip A. Rozario and Elizabeth Palley addresses long-term care policy by examining programs funded by the U.S. Administration on Aging, as well as Medicaid Waiver Programs, that support family caregiving efforts. In so doing, the authors also focus on the role of family caregiver organizations in influencing national policy to support the efforts of family caregivers in providing support for in-home and community-based resources.

Two articles in this volume focus on the increased emphasis on community-based care in the Canadian health care delivery system. An article by Pierre-Gerlier Forest and Howard A. Palley examines Canada's policy of fiscal federalism and its interplay with provincial efforts regarding regionalization and community-based health care initiatives in various Canadian provinces. The goal of such policies generally is to provide more cost-effective programs as well as a higher quality of health care in Canada's provincial health care systems. In their article, Forest and Palley deal, in part, with the experience of Quebec's Centres Locaux des Services Communitaires (CLSCs)–integrated local health and social service programs. This paper is followed by an article by Benoît Gaumer and Marie-Josée Fleury examining the history, politics and operation of CLSCs. The CLSCs provide an excellent example of a network of community-based programs integrating health and social services and often providing a team approach to the delivery of community-based health and health-related services. Under a recent Quebec reform, general hospitals, CLSCs and long-term care centers have now been merged into a new organizational form known as a Centre de Santé et des Services Sociaux (CSSS). In part, this new reform seeks greater vertical integration of local health and social services.

Next, Cheryl A. Hyde presents an excellent case study of the Womancare Health Center and the challenges it has faced in seeking to provide women's health services in an atmosphere of intimidation and harassment of its providers and patients. Hyde describes its strategy of expanding health services for women at the community-level as a means of developing community support in spite of ideologically-based anti-abortion and anti-contraception mobilization resulting in legislative constraint and community-based assaults on its ability to deliver needed health care services. Finally, another perspective on advisory committee involvement, that included the participation of consumer and provider groups, in the development of Managed Care Organizations in Medicaid programs in Connecticut is provided by Colleen M. Grogan and Michael K. Gusmano. They provide an excellent evaluation of the effectiveness of advisory committee participation and the need for more open public forum discussion by such advisory groups.

PACE:
Has It Changed
the Chronic Care Paradigm?

Marty Lynch
Mauro Hernandez
Carroll Estes

INTRODUCTION

The Program of All-inclusive Care for the Elderly (PACE) is an excellent example of an innovation developed by a local community that has had significant national policy implications. PACE was first developed by On Lok, a San Francisco elder-serving agency in Chinatown which had introduced adult day health care and wished to create a more comprehensive service to deal with the lack of skilled nursing beds appropriate to the local community (Bodenheimer, 1999). Since that time, PACE has become a Medicare benefit and parts of the model have been adopted by many state Medicaid agencies and other types of organizations interested in chronic care service delivery. To date, PACE replications have been sponsored by other non-profit organizations many of them, like On Lok, relatively small community-based groups. We will describe PACE and selected program-related findings reported in the literature, as well as discuss policy implications in a number of key chronic care areas. In addition, we include a case study describing the development of the Center for Elders Independence (CEI), a PACE site developed by a free-standing non-profit organization in Oakland California, and its impact on the local community.

METHODS

The authors completed a review of PACE relevant literature and conducted interviews with several key informants to identify important issues related to policy implications of the PACE program. Articles and reports were identified following title and keyword internet searches of databases such as PubMed and Social Science Citation Index, government websites, such as the Centers for Medicare and Medicaid Services, and the National PACE Association's website (NPA, 2004). Since the paper is not intended to be a comprehensive review of the PACE literature, the authors selected a number of articles and reports that describe important policy, relevant findings, and program characteristics for integrating health and social services for the elderly. The case study on a local PACE program was developed based on an interview with Peter Szutu, CEO of the Center for Elders Independence, and one of the authors who is a founding Board member of CEI.

WHAT WE KNOW ABOUT PACE

The Program of All-inclusive Care for the Elderly (PACE) has approximately twenty years of experience fully integrating medical and home and community-based care in a small managed care model for elders with severe chronic conditions (Eng, Pedulla, Eleazer, McCann, & Fox, 1997). Prepaid financing maximizes the flexibility needed to redesign what is otherwise a fragmented and poorly coordinated service delivery system, while risk adjustment mechanisms respond to actual costs of care for target populations (Master & Eng, 2001). Historically, PACE sites received much of their initial development capital from large national foundations. More recently developed programs have emerged from within existing hospital, health care, or long-term care systems that have the necessary resources to support start up costs (Gross, Temkin-Greener, Kunitz, & Mukamel, 2004).

Participant and Program Characteristics

All PACE participants must meet nursing home admission requirements in their state and thus have significant functional Activity of Daily Living (ADL) problems as well as several chronic disease problems. Participants must be at least 55 years old and are generally dually eligible for Medicaid and Medicare. The typical PACE participant is an 80-year old woman who is dependent in three activities of daily living (ADL) and has 8 medical diagnoses. About half of PACE participants have been diagnosed with dementia and most (95%) are Medicaid eligible (Gross et al., 2004; National PACE Association). Once enrolled, participants receive intensive care coordination provided by a multidisciplinary team that includes the PACE primary care physician, social worker, physical, speech, and occupational therapists, as well as nursing, activity and transportation staff (Shannon & Van Reenen, 1998; Zimmerman, Pemberton, & Thomas, 1998). Most PACE members attend an adult day health center co-located with a primary care clinic and receive the majority of their medical and community-based services in that setting. Depending on individual needs and preferences, additional in-home services may include skilled nursing, personal care, and other household tasks (Gross et al., 2004).

PACE programs typically contract with outside entities for hospital and medical specialty services but retain control of utilization of these services through primary care physician management. Medical providers may have special training in geriatric care or may be internists. PACE programs use information systems, which allow them to gather extensive utilization data on the full range of services provided, manage their costs, and compare themselves to other PACE programs. Some PACE programs are experimenting with electronic medical records (Szutsu, 2001).

Payment incentives in the PACE program support coordination of care and substitution of primary and basic home and community care for high cost acute and institutional care. PACE programs are required to provide basic Medicare and Medicaid services but may also choose to use other less typical interventions (Eng et al., 1997). One PACE program takes its members on fishing trips and has a small drama group, which performs at local events (Szutsu, 2001). PACE programs often are able to avoid or shorten hospital stays by substituting intensive services from the rest of the team in place of hospital care (Eng et al., 1997).

To survive financially PACE programs must manage utilization across a range of hospital, long term care, and specialty services. Although combined capitation payments from Medicare and Medicaid are relatively large, care requirements are also heavy. As noted above, PACE programs have great flexibility in funding educational or preventive activities. They are able to make decisions based on the individual patient's care plan and overall budget constraints. Given the broad range of medical and long term care risk accepted by PACE programs, they manage greater numbers of dollars per member than most managed care programs and have additional flexibility to fund preventive or community-based interventions (Eng et al., 1997).

PACE programs make efforts to involve their members and family members in the care planning and coordination process. Some PACE programs continue to use family members as caregivers for enrollees. Both physical and cognitive disabilities are significant in PACE programs and may make participant empowerment a challenge (Branch, Coulam, & Zimmerman, 1995).

Selected Outcomes

Reported positive outcomes include, "steady census growth, good consumer satisfaction, reduction in use of institutional care, controlled utilization of medical services, and cost savings to public and private payers of care, including Medicare and Medicaid." (Eng et al., 1997). Although all PACE members require a skilled nursing facility level of care, PACE programs have been able to provide hospital days per thousand at the level of the general Medicare population, as well as lower short term hospital utilization (Wieland et al., 2000). Looking at the impact of PACE on health service utilization and other outcome measures, one study finds that PACE enrollees, compared with people who decline to enroll, have: lower rates of nursing home utilization and in-patient hospitalization, higher utilization of ambulatory services, better health status and quality of life, and less physical function deterioration. PACE participation was also found to be associated with lower mortality rates (Chatterji, Burstein, Kidder, & White, 1998). In a sample of older participants from eight PACE sites, black patients, who were younger and more disabled, had lower mortality rates than white patients. This survival advantage for black patients emerged after being enrolled in PACE for one year and may be due to improved access to care compared to white patients who may have had better access prior to enrollment (Tan, Lui, Eng, Jha, & Covinsky, 2003). Compared to the general population of older decedents, PACE participants are twice as likely to die at home and half as likely to die in a hospital (Temkin-Greener & Mukamel, 2002).

Nevertheless, questions remain about effectiveness. At times PACE programs are accused of creaming or enrolling less disabled and less costly members, which may mean excluding elders with psychiatric or substance abuse problems (Branch et al., 1995; Holtzman, Chen, & Kane, 1998). Implementation of the PACE model and program characteristics are believed to be uneven as evidenced by reported variation in service utilization, changing disability rates, hospitalization rates and risks among sites (Branch et al., 1995; Mukamel, Temkin-Greener, & Clark, 1998; Wieland et al., 2000). Other reported differences by PACE site have included end of life service utilization (Mukamel, Bajorska, & Temkin-Greener, 2002), care quality (Pacala, Kane, Atherly,

& Smith, 2000), and place of death (Temkin-Greener & Mukamel, 2002).

PACE programs have successfully integrated medical and chronic care for those who choose to enroll and most PACE programs have successfully managed a very complex package of care within their budgets (Eng et al., 1997). PACE has become a recognized Medicare benefit in the Balanced Budget Act of 1997 and continues to grow, albeit at a slower rate than anticipated (Gross et al., 2004; Irvin, Massey, & Dorsey, 1997). PACE is also subject to state to state variations based on individual states' willingness to process PACE applications or negotiate the Medicaid portion of the capitation payment, given concerns about the high cost of providing the benefit. Despite these issues, PACE continues to be one of the few successful models for integrating the full range of medical and chronic care services across both the Medicare and Medicaid programs.

WHY ARE THERE ONLY 10,000 PACE PARTICIPANTS AND 32 SITES?

Slow growth, only 10,000 to 15,000 members nationwide and 32 fully capitated sites as of April, 2005, has limited the impact and significance of the PACE program (Branch et al., 1995; Kane, Illston, & Miller, 1992). PACE programs have only grown at a rate of one to four per year since the federal cap was expanded in 1997 from 16 to 40 programs upon enactment of the Balanced Budget Act, which allowed an annual increase of 20 more programs thereafter (Gross et al., 2004). There has been a limited amount of research on barriers to expansion of PACE. Gross and colleagues (2004) identified a number of barriers to PACE program growth based on 27 site visits and numerous interviews with PACE program management and staff. Interviews with PACE program administrators and staff revealed 16 barriers to participant enrollment growth, which were then ranked using scores from a follow-up survey. Although the importance of the identified barriers varied considerably by program administrator, the top five ranked barriers had to do with: (1) competition for potential disabled members from other state funded home and community-based service (HCBS) programs, (2) competition from operating in a service-rich health care environment where potential members can get their home and community service needs met elsewhere, (3) client unwillingness to give up their primary care physician, (4) out-of-pocket costs for non-Medicaid enrollment, and (5) a lack of understanding about services and eligibility among gatekeepers (Gross et al., 2004). At the federal level, they also reported the inability of potential PACE providers to predict future revenues because of new risk-adjusted Medicare payment provisions that were not made public until 2003. State efforts have also varied considerably given the substantial political will and resources needed to enable PACE program growth by making any necessary legislative or regulatory changes required to contract with additional PACE sites and developing necessary systems for information management, payment, oversight and quality assurance of PACE.

Rural location may also present a barrier for growth. To date, no PACE programs have emerged in rural areas, which tend to have a higher proportion of older residents (Fitzgerald, Morgan, & Morris, 2004). Gross and colleagues (2004) discuss how the program's reliance on day center attendance may be impractical in areas with lower population density and transportation barriers are more challenging in bringing members to service locations and getting home care workers to members' homes. The authors report that states with PACE programs average about five times as many persons per square mile as those that do not. As a result, the National PACE Association and the National Rural Health Association received federal funding to explore the modification and development of PACE in rural areas (HRSA, 2004).

In addition to reviewing available literature, we interviewed a number of key informants to provide additional insights on the issue of slow PACE growth. Informants included program administrators, researchers, and regulators familiar with PACE and other home and community-based service models. There were a number of similarities in the issues we identified but also a number of differences. The key question is: "If PACE has indeed inspired many efforts to successfully integrate acute and long term care services as well as the use of at-risk capitated financing from both Medicare and Medicaid, why does the program continue to be so small after twenty years of development?" This is a major question given the apparent promise of PACE. The answers can be classified in a number of ways.

1. *The PACE service package is not attractive to all elders.* Jenny Chin Hansen, long time CEO of On Lok, has often said that PACE is not for everyone and that we need to develop other integrated models of long term care. To date, PACE has most often relied on adult day health care services as the core of the services package. Not all potential participants want to come into a group setting

several days a week to receive their care. Some PACE programs are now experimenting with service models that are less reliant on adult day health care, shifting most service delivery to the client's home. It is thought that a number of disabled elders choose not to enroll in PACE programs because they may not wish to give up their primary care physician or to use an adult day health center approach to care, preferring instead to receive needed services at home (Kane et al., 1992). As staff-model organizations, PACE sites generally require participants to replace their current primary care and other health care providers with those employed or otherwise specified by the PACE program (Gross et al., 2004). PACE has operated like a closed-panel HMO requiring participants to give up their own physician and use a PACE staff physician when joining the program. Medicare regulations have recently been loosened to allow PACE programs to contract out medical services and some sites have accommodated member preferences through arrangements with client physicians on a fee-for-service, contract, or partnership basis. (Bodenheimer, 1999)

2. *Lack of start-up capital.* Non-profit providers lack the resources to quickly expand existing and new PACE sites. PACE programs are often sponsored by non-profits in local communities (see Figure 1, CEI case study). The very aspect that makes them part of their community fabric and community development efforts, limits their expansion. Not only are providers often associated with a local area, but non-profits typically have a hard time putting up start-up capital for significant expansion efforts. Some of the smaller non-profits may also lack the administrative infrastructure to support expanded development beyond their immediate community. In the absence of federal, state, or private grants, new programs must be able to secure financial support from a sponsoring organization that can cover startup and initial operating costs.

3. *The risk is too high for for-profits.* For-profit providers have not chosen to enter the market although 10 are permitted on a demonstration basis (Gross et al., 2004). Government regulations particularly in regard to rate setting are changing, creating potentially significant unknowns in terms of the business model of PACE. Few for-profit insurers and providers have become comfortable with the dual eligible (Medicare-Medicaid) market, nor are they familiar with the level of risk involved for the nursing home certifiable population. The tight operating margins experienced

by current PACE sites may not leave room for paying down debt while providing the required return on investment.

4. *Potential enrollees are not generally well-informed.* Significant marketing needs to take place to expose elders and their families to a relatively unknown concept of elder care. PACE availability in relatively few communities plus limited advertising budgets among the non-profit sponsors have meant that there is limited public knowledge of the product and its benefits.

5. *State political support may be constrained.* State Medicaid agencies have slowed enrollment of new PACE programs due to budget restrictions and fear that some elders who use PACE would never have really entered a nursing home (the so-called wood-work effect), therefore driving up state costs. For example California, home to four PACE sites, has placed a moratorium on processing new PACE site applications or applications for expansion of geographic service areas by existing sites, ostensibly because of lack of staff to process the applications. Home and community-based waiver programs which already exist also often compete with rather than co-operate with PACE programs (Gross et al., 2004).

6. *Medicare Advantage regulations are prohibitive.* PACE regulations are modeled on Medicare Advantage regulations for much larger managed care plans. They create a significant barrier for the types of non-profit organizations that have sponsored PACE sites to-date. To date, larger Medicare Advantage health plans have not seen the benefit of sponsoring their own PACE programs or cooperating with existing PACE sites. It is also possible that PACE regulations, such as those limiting programs' ability to contract with outside primary care physicians, may have been written before the PACE program itself had fully evolved, therefore codifying practices that were still not developed to allow future growth.

7. *Access for middle-income seniors is limited.* Frail Medicare-only clients, who represent the majority of individuals who would meet PACE's functional eligibility criteria, must "spend down" their assets in order to become eligible for Medicaid and afford PACE (Bodenheimer, 1999). Recognizing that PACE may be unaffordable to middle-income elders at risk of nursing home placement, the need for an affordable premium schedule has been widely recognized (Master & Eng, 2001). Out-of-PACE pocket costs are otherwise too high for attracting a larger segment of the frail, older population. Several PACE sites have attempted to develop products for non-Medicaid elders but have had limited success.

BROADER POLICY IMPLICATIONS OF PACE

We will examine several key PACE implications for broader policy development. PACE has already achieved an important impact by mov-

FIGURE 1. Case Study: Center for Elders Independence

CEI provides an example of a PACE site developed by a local community. CEI owes its genesis to a community forum in the mid-1980s when three Oakland, California based community organization agreed to come together to form the Coalition for Elders Independence (later renamed the Center for.....). The three included a Gray Panther founded community health center, the Over 60 Health Center (now called LifeLong Medical Care), an existing adult day health center, Community Adult Day Health Services, and a local economic development agency, the Spanish Speaking Unity Council. All three wanted to bring PACE to their communities and felt that working together would provide the best chance of success and avoid competing over scarce local support needed for start-up. The three organizations agreed to raise the necessary start-up capital of about $1 million (at that time—substantially more now) from local foundations. Other organizational problems caused the economic development agency to drop out of the process before implementation. The two remaining organizations agreed that the adult day health center would provide the first center and recruit existing participants and the health center would provide the Chair of the Board of Directors, recruiting of appropriate patients from the health center, and as much cooperation as possible in medical staffing. CEI successfully began to provide services in 1989 and moved to full PACE status with both Medicaid and Medicare capitation in 1995. The LifeLong Medical CEO still serves as an officer of the CEI Board and the original Chair of the adult day health center board is now the CEO of the PACE program. The organizations have continued to cooperate on shared facilities, program development, and home and community-based service innovation.

CEI now serves approximately 380 participants at three PACE centers in Oakland and Berkeley, California and operates with an annual budget of about $22 million. CEI serves a low income multi-ethnic community with primary emphasis on African-Americans. All three sites are located in low income communities and are important community employers. CEI employs approximately 200 staff including aids, drivers, in-home personal assistance workers, as well as physicians, nurses, and other professionals. Many of these positions are entry level and allow for local residents to move up a career ladder in the health care industry as well as have access to health and other benefits and on-going on-the-job training. In addition, CEI has worked to employ family members of participants to provide home care since in many cases

these families were relying on income from public in-home support resources before their family member entered the PACE program. CEI sites are also attractive community facilities located in community service centers which add to overall community improvement and economic development. CEI's Board of Directors is composed exclusively of local community residents and professionals including a representative of participant's families. Control is thus local and the economic benefits of the organization are returned directly to the local community.

CEI's difficulties also illustrate some of the difficulties faced in expanding PACE in general. Start-up capital was difficult to obtain. Enrollment growth has been slow with a heavy emphasis on marketing, given the lack of familiarity with the PACE benefit among community members. Other case management programs often express competitiveness with PACE as opposed to working together. Complying with federal PACE regulations has been difficult and costly for a free standing non-profit agency that does not have a large corporate infrastructure. Standards for much larger managed care organizations with hundreds of thousands of members have been required of PACE whose census typically are a few hundred. CEI has also struggled with local state regulators who do not understand the PACE model and the mix of services provided in low income senior housing locations. The regulations themselves were written to regulate categorical programs and not suitable for integrated care models. To the regulators, these innovative program efforts have sometimes looked like unlicensed nursing homes rather than alternatives that allow disabled elders to remain in the community. Battles over appropriate application of regulation are both immediately costly and require significant advocacy efforts as well. For the past year, CEI and other California PACE programs have been working with the state to modify existing state regulations to be more appropriate for integrated systems of care.

CEI is an excellent example of a local organization building service innovation as well as providing significant community development opportunities in its community. CEI was willing to take significant financial and organizational risk because of its belief in the value of the service model for low income disabled seniors. It could also apply significant sweat equity and raise some philanthropic resources without having to be concerned about a fairly short turnaround on return on investment.

ing from a locally based service and financing innovation to a standard Medicare benefit. In addition, PACE has influenced the development of State Medicaid and long term care programs and may have implications for the Medicare Advantage managed care program and private long term care insurance development.

PACE Innovations Diffused to State Long Term Care Programs

The PACE program, as originated by On Lok, was one of the first efforts to integrate acute medical and chronic long term care services and to bring together Medicare and Medicaid financing streams in a single capitated funding package. This model became the inspiration for a number of creative efforts to accomplish integration of medical and long term care on a larger scale. Many states efforts to develop model programs for their aged and disabled populations stem from On Lok's successful experience in caring for a very disabled elderly population in an integrated format. Several states have established initiatives which attempt to integrate medical and chronic long term care for their Medicare-Medicaid eligible population in single health plans (Coleman, Grothaus, Sandhu, & Wagner, 1999; National Chronic Care Consortium, 2001). Financial and operational integration for these programs is difficult without a Medicare waiver given beneficiaries' ability to freely choose to either enroll in a managed care plan or remain in traditional fee-for-service Medicare (Wiener & Stevenson, 1998). Several states have been able to secure Medicare waivers and thus integrate financing streams as PACE does. Others have enrolled dual eligibles into Medicaid managed care programs and attempted to coordinate services by having contracting health plans receive Medicare funds in a separate but parallel funding stream to Medicaid dollars. Many of these plans also attempt to use some variation of the multi-disciplinary team emphasized by PACE to manage care for participants. A number of the state efforts place health plans at financial risk through monthly per member payment systems. PACE alone has emphasized the use of Adult Day Health Care as a focal point for delivery of a wide range of health, socialization, and therapy services.

Minnesota, Massachusetts, and Wisconsin have all secured Medicare waivers to pursue an integrated financing approach. The State of Minnesota established the Minnesota Senior Health Options (MSHO) in 1997 for frail, older dual-eligibles and the Minnesota Disability Health Options (MnDHO) program in 2002 for individuals with disabilities (Ryan & Super, 2003). Both programs allow Medicaid funds to be blended with Medicare dollars through a Medicare waiver allowing health plans to integrate delivery and financing of a full range of medical and chronic long term care services in a number of health plans from which beneficiaries can choose (Parker & Maruska, 2002). MSHO includes case management services for high-risk patients, as well as financial incentives to encourage the use of home and community-based services and early nursing home discharges (Kane, Kane, & Ladd, 1998; Stone, 2000). Examining changes in functional and satisfaction measures for MSHO enrollees, families and matched controls, Kane and colleagues (Kane, Homyak, Bershadsky, Lum, & Siadaty, 2003) found few differences in functional, satisfaction, and caregiver burden outcomes.

Massachusetts has also secured a Medicare waiver to allow for the use of both Medicaid and Medicare funds for the frail population. The model uses links between Senior Care Organizations (SCOs) and medical plans to deliver a coordinated health and long term care benefit to a broader population that includes nursing home residents and community-based elderly who are less impaired (Flanders, 2003).

The Wisconsin Partnership Program is a variation of the PACE design that allows participants to continue using their primary care physician and use substantially less day care. The program began operating with a full Medicaid/Medicare capitation in 1999 and was serving 1,823 clients as of February 2005, which includes both older and younger individuals with disabilities under the age of 65 (Wisconsin Department of Health & Family Services, 2005). Findings from an evaluation of this demonstration showed that Wisconsin Partnership Program enrolled clients who were less disabled than PACE enrollees, with no significant differences in reported unmet needs or beneficiary satisfaction (Kane, Homyak, & Bershadsky, 2002). A second study comparing Wisconsin Partnership Program clients to matched controls found lower disability rates among the Wisconsin Partnership Program sample and few differences in unmet needs or satisfaction (Kane, Homyak, Bershadsky, & Lum, 2002).

A number of other states (Florida, Texas, Oregon, etc.) have established initiatives for the elderly using mechanisms such as Medicaid Home and Community-Based Waiver programs (Coleman, 1998; Mollica & Riley, 1997). Texas Star Plus uses concurrent Medicaid 1915(b) and 1915(c) waivers to provide acute and long term care services to disabled and elderly Medicaid beneficiaries with Medicare enrollment in one of the participating plans being voluntary with an enriched benefit structure serving as an incentive. These programs typically rely on care coordination services to achieve integration between acute and long-term care services (Wiener & Stevenson, 1998) and do not attempt to formally integrate Medicare financing with Medicaid.

In all of these state-based efforts, providers may attempt to improve care by using chronic disease management protocols (Lynch, Estes, & Hernandez, 2003a), but the main intervention is the effort to integrate acute medical and chronic long term care services through the combined use of Medicare for acute and primary-care services and Medicaid for home and community-based care services, often with a case manager helping facilitate the care (Mollica & Riley, 1997). Likewise, the level of utilization and management procedures will depend on whether the participating plan or provider is at risk for the whole range of services, such as in the PACE program, or only for Medicaid services if dual eligible beneficiaries do not choose to enroll in the same Medicare plan, thus splitting the financing for medical and long term care services. Although the state demonstrations which operate without Medicare waivers attempt to align incentives between the Medicare and Medicaid programs, for the most part there remain perverse incentives for states to maximize expenditures borne by the Medicare program and for Medicare providers to shift costs to Medicaid (Wiener & Stevenson, 1998). For example, Medicaid reimbursed nursing homes may have little incentive to manage acute episodes of chronic conditions inhouse, rather than simply sending the resident to the hospital, which will be covered by Medicare. States may also require nursing homes to become certified under Medicare as well as Medicaid in order to shift some costs to Medicare (Mollica & Riley, 1997; Wiener & Stevenson, 1998).

In addition to perverse financial incentives for the state plans that do not secure Medicare waivers, it is also difficult for such programs to secure the same level of day to day service coordination that PACE achieves. Difficulties in achieving continuity of care arise when medical services are provided by a different organization than the provider of home and community-services and when care coordination or case management functions may be co-located with one of these two or in a third organization. Although the goal of these programs may be consistent with the integration of care for the patient as in the PACE model, it is difficult to achieve when services are sponsored by different organizations housed in different locations. It is also unclear whether such "less integrated" plans will be able to achieve the level of utilization control for hospital and nursing home days achieved by PACE (Chatterji et al.,

1998; Wieland et al., 2000). It may be more difficult to bring to bear the full range of home and community resources for members experiencing acute medical problems when home and community providers are not part of the medical management team.

Although state sponsored programs have used and adapted PACE related innovations, they remain significantly different in many ways. These include level of integration; inclusiveness of the multi-disciplinary team; how financial incentives are aligned; and whether or not Medicare financing is fully integrated with Medicaid funds. In addition, although many states provide reimbursement for adult day health care (Lucas, Rosato, Lee, & Howell-White, 2002), the use of ADHC as the focal point for service delivery and coordination seems to be a unique feature of PACE programs.

Medicare Advantage

Medicare managed care programs now referred to as Medicare Advantage have taken a number of steps to manage chronic disease. These actions have fallen into two types of activity. The first include a range of disease management programs (Lynch et al., 2003a) which focus on a specific disease entity such as diabetes, provide evidence based protocols and information support to providers, and at the same time educate patients about their health, and engage them in a more active way in the care process. The second include a range of case management programs which may work to control utilization, educate the patient, and/or coordinate other benefits (Boult, Rassen, Rassen, Moore, & Robison, 2000; Chen, Brown, Aliotta, & Fox, 2000). For the most part, these chronic care related programs have not focused on integrating home and community-based services for disabled or frail members. An exception was the Social Health Maintenance Organization demonstration (Wooldridge et al., 2001), which specifically included a limited long term care benefit in a Medicare managed care structure.

Little is known about the potential for partnerships between mainstream Medicare health plans and PACE programs given the relatively limited linkages to date. It is possible that PACE programs, which serve only a nursing home certifiable population, could take on and provide care for that very frail part of an HMO's membership. It is also possible that Medicare Advantage plans, or the so-called Special Needs Plans (SNP) authorized by the Medicare Modernization Act, could learn from PACE's multi-disciplinary approach and ability to substitute primary geriatric care, home, and community services for acute hospital care.

PACE clearly has also been successful in aligning financial incentives to support that substitution. A sophisticated PACE plan may also apply to operate a Special Needs Plan authorized under Medicare Advantage and serve a broader population. A PACE program working in partnership with an HMO or several HMOs could also successfully provide management of disabled elderly members who wish to remain in the community. Willingness to allow PACE programs to work with non-staff physician models would also facilitate such partnerships. Medicare Advantage programs may also be able to learn from PACE about management of multiple medical and disability problems since the average PACE member has 8 medical conditions (National PACE Association, 2003). This very complex, functionally disabled population is one which Medicare managed care organizations have had less comfort and experience with and may be able to learn from PACE's successes. The Medicare Advantage program, if nothing else, will incentivize more elders to join managed care plans and may, once again, make the concept of managed care more acceptable, thus supporting growth of and experimentation with PACE related models.

Private Long Term Care Insurance

PACE programs have typically been sponsored by non-profit organizations that are rooted in the communities they serve. The private long term care insurance industry would appear to be the antithesis of PACE with its sponsorship by large corporate insurance companies. Yet both have a shared interest in reducing nursing home utilization and maximizing the ability of beneficiaries to remain in the community. Nonetheless, the movement of the industry away from an emphasis on nursing home coverage towards a product which can be used to support stays in the community, is following the same trend that PACE so elegantly symbolizes. Consumers have clearly stated their desire to avoid nursing homes if at all possible. Much of PACE's popularity stems from its ability to take a population, which by all health and disability standards, qualifies for nursing home care, and help its members successfully remain in the community. As such it has inspired most of the current models of home and community-based service delivery. Despite PACE's influence in changing the paradigm of integrated chronic care, there has been little cross fertilization between PACE and long term care insurance. A few PACE programs have discussed making PACE a benefit that can be substituted for nursing home care in a long term care insurance product but there is no data yet available on these efforts. Insofar as PACE provides one more option for insurers to offer, and their liability and risk is capped to a certain set payment, there may be additional experimentation in this area.

Political Economy Issues

In our past work, we have been interested in understanding who stands to gain or lose as a result of certain policy options. Corporate U.S. interests have a major stake in both the financing and delivery of long term care services. Like other health services, long term care as a formal service delivery system (excluding the large proportion of informal unpaid care rendered by family caregivers) is organized and provided in ways that are congruent with the dominant market ideology of U.S. society. Many long term care services are provided on a proprietary basis and available primarily to those who can pay for them privately. From the political economy perspective, long term care provision is consistent with existing structural realities. It is partially state-supported, but reinforces an ideology consistent with a market approach. What does this mean? Long term care is delivered in a way that supports opportunities for profits to be made from its delivery; it involves finance capital through the insurance, pharmaceutical and other industries; and it reinforces the concept of private versus public responsibility (Ehrenreich & Ehrenreich, 1978).

The relative underdevelopment of community-based long term care, including the slow growth of PACE, falls within this larger political and economic context. Such services do not develop in a vacuum and the policies shaping these services reflect a broader structural reality. Economic, political and socio-cultural factors have influenced the development of long term care systems in the United States and to a great extent delineated future directions of policy, financing, and service delivery development.

Efforts to encourage the purchase of long term care from private insurers are consistent with the U.S. market ideology that individuals should take financial responsibility for their own health and long term care needs in ways that bolster a profitable private insurance industry. An emphasis on private insurance solutions has the benefit for corporations of reducing public pressure for a publicly financed system of long term care (as a right or entitlement) which might drain more of corporate profits into taxes and divert resources from the profitable private insurance industry. Despite the exceedingly small number of firms who offer any long term care benefits, for the most part corporate interests have resisted taking any direct responsibility for long term care costs. Corporations have allowed the state to take responsibility for the poorest needing long term care through the Medicaid program and to shunt the remaining burden to the individuals and family caregivers (often women). Near-poor elders needing long term care, particularly those most exploited during their working years, women and minorities and those living alone, are often left to fend for themselves. The result is a two-tier or two-class welfare state in which the poor receive benefits through state-variable Medicaid and other programs, while the non-poor either pay privately or, in a some cases, receive benefits through insurance programs.

Pressure for long term care reform through improvement and coverage of publicly supported and universally available community-based services (as offered through the PACE program) comes from progressive organizations attempting an expansion of the welfare-state function. Despite the demographic imperative and the work of advocates (e.g., Families USA, Gray Panthers, AARP), chances of any major expansion of long term care coverage at the federal government level are slim at this time (Estes, Wiener, Goldberg, & Goldensen, 2000) because of the conservatism of congress, the skyrocketing federal deficit with military and tax cut expenditures, the ratcheting down of welfare expenditures, and the relatively weak organization of advocacy, labor, and progressive political groups in the United States.

Consistent with the economic realities discussed above, the 2003 Medicare Modernization Act's move towards incentivizing beneficiaries to join private health plans and away from traditional fee-for-service Medicare can be seen as part of an effort to privatize an existing social insurance program. Privatization allows private businesses to make a profit on the delivery of what might be considered social goods and thus could be seen to benefit the insurance industry, private providers, and their financial backers over against the interest of tax payers, who may pay more, or beneficiaries who may see services restricted in order to achieve profit margins. When we examine the development of PACE through this lens, we have mixed findings. On one hand, PACE programs have been developed by community-based non-profits or non-profit health care systems. They have added to community infrastructure, become significant local employers, and provided an important model for consumers to receive chronic care services at home and in the community. On the other hand, there is nothing intrinsic about the PACE model that should prevent its adoption by for-profit sponsors and from becoming another health plan or insurance instrument as discussed above. In the past, we have commented that, "if all managed care plans for the elderly were like On Lok , managed care would be good for the elderly" (Lynch & Estes, 1997). PACE to date has presented a community and beneficiary responsive way to deliver chronic care to the elderly, but there are no protections in the model, per se, (such as community control of governing boards or prohibition of for-profits) which would prevent it from being subject to the same privatization forces as the Medicare program itself.

As noted above, the lack of for-profit PACE participation by private insurers and health plans may be partly explained by the program's perceived risks and limited profitability. As additional for-profit providers like Evercare, a subsidiary of United Health Care Group (Ryan & Super, 2003) become familiar with managing complex dual eligible elders, there is no reason to believe that they won't also enter the PACE market with the concomitant benefits to the private sector and potential risks to the public and consumers.

Consumer Empowerment

The authors have also examined chronic care models from the point of view of consumer control and empowerment (Lynch et al., 2003a; Lynch, Estes, & Hernandez, 2003b). PACE has potential strengths in this area. In so far as the multi-disciplinary team works with participants and their families to develop a care plan that fits the patients needs and preferences, PACE can develop a very consumer-friendly approach to care with significantly more patient control available than in most institutional or fractured models. At the same time, there are several factors which must be guarded against. PACE is an adult day health centered model. Some participants may prefer more of a home-based model. PACE financial incentives and model design may mitigate against meeting individual preferences in this area. In addition, adult day health centers may or may not include activities that allow participants to interact with their world and community in a meaningful way. PACE has made efforts to assure meaningful activities for participants. Undoubtedly there is additional progress that could be made involving participants in budgeting for their own care and understanding the financial constraints of the model. In so far as the model is community-based, offers a full range of services, and is incentivized to keep users at home, our judgment is that is a relatively consumer friendly model of chronic care with potential for consumer and family empowerment.

CONCLUSIONS

PACE demonstrates the potential of locally developed models of home and community care alternatives. In addition to significant community development and service benefits to the localities which are home to PACE programs and their members, there have clearly also been benefits to national and state policy development. PACE has been a key force in building a new paradigm supporting the value of integrated chronic care services and financing which emphasizes functional status over a strict medical model. PACE continues to be one of the few successful, although small, models that provides an alternative to nursing homes and as such has fostered a number of innovations in Medicare and Medicaid policy. Changes in the financing of PACE to include non-Medicaid populations, flexibility in the model itself, increased sophistication in marketing approaches, state-level support, and more appropriate federal regulation will all be required if PACE is to grow significantly and become an even more important influence on long term care policy and delivery for the baby boom generation quickly approaching old age. Master and Eng (2001) suggest that PACE does not represent a new system breakthrough or invention but a successful application of what advocates, policymakers and clinicians have proposed for decades. The authors disagree and believe that PACE has significantly influenced our paradigm and vision of what community-based long term care could be through its success in breaking down silos and integrating services and dollars. Unfortunately, the limited number of members in PACE compromises the ability of this primarily community-oriented model to meet its promise and bring about real structural change in a long term care system which continues to be dominated, in total societal dollars spent, by for-profit nursing homes that are almost universally feared by the elderly and disabled. PACE has played a key role in placing community-based long term care onto the policy map and establishing the value of integrated care and financing. It has a long way to go before we can say that it has really changed our overall approach to long term care from an institutional base to the community.

REFERENCES

Bodenheimer, T. (1999). Long-term care for frail elderly people–the On Lok model. *New England Journal of Medicine, 341*(17), 1324-1328.

Boult, C., Rassen, J., Rassen, A., Moore, R. J., & Robison, S. (2000). The effect of case management on the costs of health care for enrollees in Medicare Plus Choice plans: A randomized trial. *Journal of the American Geriatric Society, 48*(8), 996-1001.

Branch, L. G., Coulam, R. F., & Zimmerman, Y. A. (1995). The PACE evaluation: Initial findings. *Gerontologist, 35*(3), 349-359.

Chatterji, P., Burstein, N., Kidder, D., & White, A. (1998). *Evaluation of the Program of All-Inclusive Care for the Elderly (PACE) Demonstration: The Impact of PACE on participant Outcomes.* Washington, DC: HCFA Office of Strategic Planning.

Chen, A., Brown, R., Aliotta, S., & Fox, P. D. (2000). *Best Practices in Coordinated Care* (Contract No.: HCFA 500-95-0048 (04); MPR Reference No.: 8534-004). Princeton, NJ: Mathematica Policy Research.

Coleman, B. (1998). *New directions for state long-term care systems: Second edition* (98-09). Washington, DC: AARP Public Policy Insititute.

Coleman, E. A., Grothaus, L. C., Sandhu, N., & Wagner, E. H. (1999). Chronic care clinics: A randomized controlled trial of a new model of primary care for frail older adults. *Journal of the American Geriatric Society, 47*(7), 775-783.

Ehrenreich, J., & Ehrenreich, B. (1978). Medicine and social control. In J. Ehrenreick (Ed.), *The cultural crisis of modern medicine* (pp. 29-79). New York: Monthly Review Press.

Eng, C., Pedulla, J., Eleazer, G. P., McCann, R., & Fox, N. (1997). Program of All-inclusive Care for the Elderly (PACE): An innovative model of integrated geriatric care and financing. *Journal of the American Geriatric Society, 45*(2), 223-232.

Estes, C. L., Wiener, J. M., Goldberg, S. C., & Goldensen, S. M. (2000). The politics of long term care reform under the Clinton health plan: Lessons for the future. In P. R. Lee & C. L. Estes (Eds.), *The Nation's Health* (6th ed., pp. 206-214). Boston, MA: Jones & Bartlett.

Fitzgerald, P., Morgan, A., & Morris, T. (2004). Rural policy development: An NRHA and PACE association collaborative model. *Journal of Rural Health, 20*(1), 92-96.

Flanders, D. (2003, November 21). *MassHealth Senior Care Options.* Available: www. hhp.umd.edu/AGING/MMIP/sandiegoflanders.HTML [2003, Dec. 12].

Gross, D. L., Temkin-Greener, H., Kunitz, S., & Mukamel, D. B. (2004). The Growing Pains of Integrated Health Care for the Elderly: Lessons from the Expansion of PACE. *Milbank Quarterly, 82*(2), 257-282.

Holtzman, J., Chen, Q., & Kane, R. (1998). The effect of HMO status on the outcomes of home-care after hospitalization in a Medicare population. *Journal of the American Geriatric Society, 46*(5), 629-634.

HRSA. (2004). *Rural PACE.* U.S. Department of Health and Human Services, Health Resources and Services Administration (HRSA). Available: http://ruralhealth.hrsa. gov/pace [2005].

Irvin, C. V., Massey, S., & Dorsey, T. (1997). Determinants of enrollment among applicants to PACE. *Health Care Finance Review, 19*(2), 135-153.

Kane, R. A., Kane, R. L., & Ladd, R. C. (1998). *The Heart of Long-Term Care.* New York: Oxford University Press.

Kane, R. L., Homyak, P., & Bershadsky, B. (2002). Consumer reactions to the Wisconsin Partnership Program and its parent, the Program for All-Inclusive Care of the Elderly (PACE). *Gerontologist, 42*(3), 314-320.

Kane, R. L., Homyak, P., Bershadsky, B., & Lum, Y. S. (2002). Consumer responses to the Wisconsin Partnership Program for Elderly Persons: a variation on the PACE Model. *Journal of Gerontology: Series A Biological Sciences and Medical Sciences, 57*(4), M250-258.

Kane, R. L., Homyak, P., Bershadsky, B., Lum, Y. S., & Siadaty, M. S. (2003). Outcomes of managed care of dually eligible older persons. *Gerontologist, 43*(2), 165-174.

Kane, R. L., Illston, L. H., & Miller, N. A. (1992). Qualitative analysis of the Program of All-inclusive Care for the Elderly (PACE). *Gerontologist, 32*(6), 771-780.

Lucas, J. A., Rosato, N. S., Lee, J. A., & Howell-White, S. (2002). *Adult Day Health Services: A Review of the Literature.* Trenton, NJ: Rutgers Center for State Health Policy, Rutgers University.

Lynch, M., & Estes, C. L. (1997). Is managed care good for older persons? In A. E. Scharlach & L. W. Kaye (Eds.), *Controversial Issues in Aging* (pp. 120-123). Boston: Allyn & Bacon.

Lynch, M., Estes, C. L., & Hernandez, M. (2003a). Chronic-Care Initiatives: What We Have Learned and Implications for the Medicare Program. *In Long Term Care and Medicare Policy: Can We Improve the Continuity of Care?* (pp. 151-174). Washington, DC: The Brookings Institution and National Academy of Social Insurance.

Lynch, M., Estes, C. L., & Hernandez, M. (2003b). Consumer empowerment issues in chronic and long-term care. In P. Lee & C. L. Estes (Eds.), *The Nation's Health* (7th ed., pp. 579-587). Sudbury, MA: Jones & Bartlett.

Master, R. J., & Eng, C. (2001). Integrating acute and long-term care for high-cost populations. *Health Affairs, 20*(6), 161-172.

Mollica, R., & Riley, T. (1997). *Managed Care for Low Income Elders Dually Eligible for Medicaid and Medicare: A Snapshot of State and Federal Activity.* Portland, Maine: National Academy for State Health Policy.

Mukamel, D. B., Bajorska, A. M., & Temkin-Greener, H. P. (2002). Health Care Services Utilization at the End of Life in a Managed Care Program Integrating Acute and Long-Term Care. *Medical Care, 40*(12), 1136-1148.

Mukamel, D. B., Temkin-Greener, H., & Clark, M. L. (1998). Stability of disability among PACE enrollees: Financial and programmatic implications. *Health Care Financing Review, 19*(3), 83-100.

National Chronic Care Consortium. (2001). *Primary Care for People with Chronic Conditions: Issues and Models. A Technical Assistance Paper of The Robert Wood Johnson Foundation Medicare/Medicaid Integration Program*: University of Maryland Center on Aging.

National PACE Association. (2003). *Who does PACE serve?* Available: http://www.npaonline.org/website/article.asp?id=50 [2005, Feb. 3].

NPA. (2004). *Bibliography of PACE-Related Articles*. National PACE Association (NPA). Available: http://www.npaonline.org/website/article.asp?id=63 [2005, January 31].

Pacala, J. T., Kane, R. L., Atherly, A. J., & Smith, M. A. (2000). Using structured implicit review to assess quality of care in the Program of All-Inclusive Care for the Elderly (PACE). *Journal of the American Geriatric Society, 48*(8), 903-910.

Parker, P., & Maruska, D. (2002). *Minnesota Disability Health Options Project Summary*. Minnesota Department of Human Services. Available: http://www.dhs.state.mn.us/main/groups/healthcare/documents/pub/DHS_id_017511.pdf [2005, March 3].

Ryan, J., & Super, N. (2003). Dually eligible for Medicare and Medicaid: Two for one or double jeopardy? *Issue Brief National Health Policy Forum* (794), 1-24.

Shannon, K., & Van Reenen, C. (1998). PACE (Program of All-Inclusive Care for the Elderly): Innovative care for the frail elderly. Comprehensive services enable most participants to remain at home. *Health Progress, 79*(5), 41-45.

Stone, R. (2000). *Long Term Care for the Elderly with Disabilities: Current Policy, Emerging Trends, and Implications for the 21st Century*. Milbank Memorial Fund. Available: http://www.milbank.org/0008stone/ [2000, Dec. 5].

Szutsu, P. (2001). Personal communication with Peter Szutsu, Director, Center for Elders Independence. Oakland, CA.

Tan, E. J., Lui, L. Y., Eng, C., Jha, A. K., & Covinsky, K. E. (2003). Differences in mortality of black and white patients enrolled in the program of all-inclusive care for the elderly. *Journal of the American Geriatric Society, 51*(2), 246-251.

Temkin-Greener, H., & Mukamel, D. B. (2002). Predicting place of death in the program of all-inclusive care for the elderly (PACE): Participant versus program characteristics. *Journal of the American Geriatric Society, 50*(1), 125-135.

Wieland, D., Lamb, V. L., Sutton, S. R., Boland, R., Clark, M., Friedman, S., Brummel-Smith, K., & Eleazer, G. P. (2000). Hospitalization in the Program of All-Inclusive Care for the Elderly (PACE): Rates, concomitants, and predictors. *Journal of the American Geriatric Society, 48*(11), 1373-1380.

Wiener, J. M., & Stevenson, D. G. (1998). State policy on long-term care for the elderly. *Health Affairs, 17*(3), 81-100.

Wisconsin Department of Health & Family Services. (2005). *Wisonsin Partnership Program Census Graphs*. Available: http://www.dhfs.state.wi.us/WIpartnership/census.htm [2005, March 15].

Wooldridge, J., Brown, R., Foster, L., Hoag, S., Irvin, C., Kane, R. L., Newcomer, R., Schneider, B., & Smith, K. (2001). *Social Health Maintenance Organizations: Transition into Medicare + Choice* (Contract No. 500-96-005 (2)). Washington, DC: submitted to Health Care Financing Administration.

Zimmerman, Y. A., Pemberton, D., & Thomas, L. (1998). *Evaluation of the Program of All-Inclusive Care for the Elderly (PACE) Demonstration: Factors Contributing to Care Management and Decision Making in the PACE Model* (HCFA Contract # 500-96-0003/TO4). Washington, DC: HCFA Office of Strategic Planning.

Integrated Care: Incentives, Approaches, and Future Considerations

L. Gail Dobell

Robert J. Newcomer

INTRODUCTION

Taken together health and long term care services and practices constitute a continuum of care, but one that is highly compartmentalized. These compartments are varyingly defined: sometimes by the setting (e.g., hospital, nursing home), sometimes by the provider (e.g., primary care physician, social worker), sometimes by body system or disease (e.g., dementia, congestive heart failure), or by severity of the conditions (e.g., disability, nursing home certifiable, terminal). Compartmentalization has been reinforced and in turn has influenced the means of financing and regulating these different levels and types of care. There have been persistent demarcations between hospital and custodial nursing home care, and between nursing homes and community services. Transitions between providers and/or settings is one problematic aspect of compartmentalization. This can disrupt the "continuity of care" for individuals. Another consequence is cost shifting from one payer to another. All of these factors may contribute to a suboptimization of the delivery system's overall effectiveness.

Attempts addressing one or more facets of compartmentalization are promoted under terms like "integration of care," "continuity of care," and "continuum of care." This paper describes recent trends and approaches to integration. Our intention is to place these into the context of the points of transitions between levels of care, review the accomplishments of selected efforts, and then suggest research and policy de-velopments to further explore attainment of integrated care. Specific attention is given to disease management and other in patient and out patient initiatives, including the Program of All-Inclusive Care for the Elderly (PACE).

CONTINUUM OF HEALTH & LONG TERM CARE

Recognizing that integration has been variously defined, we begin with a framework that characterizes the continuum of health and long term services. The continuum, shown in Figure 1, is organized into three main dimensions based on health status: the absence of a condition(s) where the emphasis is on condition prevention, the presence of a condition(s) where the emphasis is on acute and chronic condition management, and finally, the Advance Illness stage where the emphasis could shift to palliative care. Shown in each status level are examples of the types of services and providers who would be involved. These areas of overlap between the health status dimensions are the opportunities for achieving care integration.

This framework is synthesized fro multiple sources: best-practices in chronic care (Reuben, 2002; Wagner, Austin et al., 2001) and disease management (Foote, 2004; Villagra, 2004), integrated care (Stone & Katz, 1996) long-term care (Wiener & Stevenson, 1998) and Medicare reform (Cassel, Besdine, & Siegel, 1999; Whitelaw & Warden, 1999).

To briefly illustrate how one might interpret the framework, consider the example of an individual having no notable health problems. The "care" needed would be a combination of prevention education, selfmanagement, and primary health care. Once diagnosed with a health condition, an individual progresses to condition management consisting of primary care, specialists, and episodic acute care. This array likely involves two or more medical providers, and others who assist in treatment adherence and self management. If physical function and/or mental or cognitive limitations are involved, then assistive and various non-

FIGURE 1. Continuum of Care

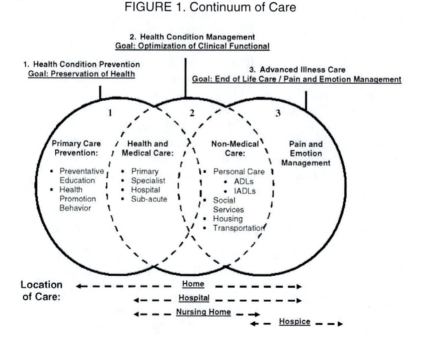

medical services may be required to facilitate activities of daily living (ADL) and instrumental activities of daily living (IADL), and social needs. Most of the condition management population resides in community settings, although a portion may be living in congregate or group settings or nursing homes. For some, communication and treatment adherence and training and support may begin to involve informal caregivers in addition to the patient or recipient. An individual's health status may progress to an end or terminal stage. As this occurs, the care could shift from active management of the health conditions to one of palliation, where the emphasis is more on symptom management, patient comfort and pain management, than on treatment. Advanced illness care is achieved through supportive assistance and modifications in medical care.

CURRENT CMS ACTIVITIES AND THE INTEGRATION OF CARE

Research and policy development and evaluation activities related to health and human services are distributed among a number of agencies within federal and state governments. The programs emphasized in the present discussion are those of Medicare and Medicaid. Both programs are administered by the Centers for Medicare & Medicaid Services (CMS). Medicare is a federal program financing hospital, physician, and other skilled health care services (e.g., home health, skilled nursing, rehabilitation) for the aged and disabled beneficiaries. Medicaid, is jointly financed by state and federal sources, and is targeted to those with low income. This program covers the health care services financed by Medicare and an array of services thought of as long term care. Among these are custodial nursing home care, home and community-based services (e.g., personal care, home maker services, adult day health care).

CMS' research and evaluation program is focused largely on the performance of its programs and the effect of policy changes on them. Many of these efforts are mandated by legislation. Consequently, CMS research and demonstration activity is a window into national policy and programs. CMS characterizes its current research activity into the eight, sometimes overlapping themes summarized in Figure 2 (CMS, 2005). We review this activity to illustrate the breadth of efforts, and to highlight gaps and assumptions about effective practices.

Vulnerable Populations. A starting point in assessing CMS efforts is recognizing that this agency's programs provide health care financing

FIGURE 2. Current CMS Research Activity Summarized by Theme

Monitoring & Evaluating CMS Programs

These efforts in combination with projects listed under other themes provide information on the infrastructure of the health system; populations of health care users; service and expenditure patterns; variations in costs, quality, and access to care; and on the effects of CMS's program changes on beneficiaries. Among active projects are several looking the effects of change in policy on managed care participation and access to post acute care benefits, like rehabilitation therapy and home health care; surveys of health plan member satisfaction and beneficiary health care knowledge; factors influencing health provider choice, including the availability of information about quality of care; and evaluation of the services and utilization under home and community care waiver program. There are three projects addressing aspects of the continuum of care. One of these examines the long term care episodes and care history of beneficiaries, another factors associated with hospitalization rates for ambulatory care sensitive conditions, and third looks at patterns of injury among beneficiaries and the consequences for cost, income, mortality and morbidity.

Strengthening Medicaid, State Children's Health Insurance Programs, & State Programs

Children and their families account for about two-thirds of population served by Medicaid (a national program combining federal and state resources directed at low income populations). The elderly and individuals with disabilities, the balance of Medicaid enrollees, account for more than two-thirds of program expenditures. Projects under this theme include a number that expand health care eligibility to cover otherwise uninsured children or to cover community based long term care services that would otherwise not be available. Commonly combined with these more flexible eligibility rule are limits on enrollment or requirements for enrollment in managed care. These projects are monitored for effects on access and utilization control. Included too are evaluations of various forms of utilization control: case management over community based long term care benefits and nursing home admission. A large number of states have demonstrations intended to increase access to community based care and as part of this effort many are attempting to "improve" the direct care workforce through recruitment, training, registries and more public information. A few states are testing consumer interest and financial costs associated with consumer-directed personal assistance workers. There are two projects (more listed under other CMS themes) that expressly integrate acute and long term care funding for the aged and those under age 65 with qualifying disabilities All enrollee must be eligible for both Medicare and Medicaid, and most meet criteria for being nursing home eligible at time of enrollment. Another integrative project is targeted solely on persons in nursing homes. Its purpose is to "manage" the acute care needs of persons in nursing homes.

Expanding Beneficiaries' Choices and Availability of Managed Care Options

The predominant activity under this theme is toward foster changes within managed care delivery systems to include Preferred Provider Organizations (PPOs) and Point of Service (POS) plans. Among others, there are projects evaluating alternative prospective payment methodologies for managed health care and diagnostic cost group risk adjustment models. There is also continuing work evaluating operations and quality assurance within the Program for All-Inclusive Care for the Elderly (PACE) and in promoting state interest in identifying additional PACE markets.

Developing Fee for Service and Service Delivery Systems

Much of the current work under this theme addresses effects of prospective payment systems (PPSs changes stipulated by the Balance Budget Act of 1997. These varyingly effect skilled nursing facilities, home health, inpatient rehabilitation, and outpatient and long-term care hospitals. Among other things these studies are looking home health case mix, post-acute care provision across alternative provider settings, access and use of rehabilitation. There are also projects supporting a Medicare Centers for Excellence Demonstration. This is illustrative of several demonstrations that align hospital and physician incentives, including all-inclusive payments for hospital and physician services for specific inpatient episodes of care. These projects are typically targeted to specific diagnoses. A number of other projects implement payment and service delivery demonstrations mandated by the Medicare Modernization Act.

FIGURE 2. (Continued)

Improving Quality of Care and Performance Under CMS Programs
Quality has been a key theme for a number of years. This has involved the development of indicators of quality as well as data systems to compile and report this information, and incentives for providers to improve quality. Generally these efforts have been focused on specific elements in the delivery system: physician group practice, hospitals, inpatient rehabilitation, nursing homes, home health, and home and community-based services. Some efforts have been even more specific to particular procedures like renal dialysis, and heart failure monitoring. Under this theme the data systems and quality monitoring processes have not extended across elements in the continuum of care.

Improving the Health of the Beneficiary Population
Six percent of Medicare beneficiaries account for 50 percent of Medicare spending. This fact has influenced CMS efforts to either identify those likely to become high risk or to more commonly to limit access to benefits to only those who meet the risk criteria. Sometimes this is a level of physical or mental frailty, sometimes the presence of a particular chronic condition. Targeting is thought to improve the cost effectiveness. One program illustrating this theme is directed to physician performance in the management of selected chronic conditions (e.g., cancer, chronic obstructive pulmonary disease, congestive heart failure, coronary artery disease, depression, diabetes) among non-institutionalized patient. This approach uses combinations of self-management and case management, sometimes combined with capitation payment. Among the goals of these programs are a reduction of preventable disability and hospital use. Hospice and Advanced Illness Coordinated Care programs and end stage renal disease management are examples of programs directed more specifically to end of life care. These too seek to reduce hospital use. Also under this theme are projects directed to revenue sources. Among these is one promoting reverse mortgages as a means to finance long term care.

Prescription Drugs
Studies are being developed to evaluate the implementation of the Medicare drug card and drug benefits. These include an examination of enrollment, prescription drug coverage estimates, and per capita spending for covered drugs. A demonstration mandated by section 641 of the Medicare Modernization Act paying for selected new drugs or biologicals will also be implemented.

Building Research Capacity
CMS supports a range of activities to build and improve our health services research capacity, both internally and externally to CMS. The intent of these efforts is to increase the efficiency of our research and demonstration program and meet the broad research needs of CMS and the wider health research community. These activities support two objectives: (1) to sponsor programs to improve the infrastructure of the U.S. health services research system, and (2) to provide tools to facilitate health services research and to support CMS's effective and efficient research program. The programs to improve the infrastructure are directed at developing or enhancing the expertise of researchers outside the Government, and they often also support broader Federal government initiatives. The tools to facilitate health services research are carried out to support CMS's own research operations as well as to provide information that benefits external health care research related to CMS's programs.

Source: This synopsis was derived from Centers for Medicare & Medicaid Services (CMS). (2005) *CMS Research Activities: The Active Projects Report.* http://www.cms.hhs.gov/researchers/projects/apr/default.asp. Refer to this web site for a complete listing of projects.

for some of the Nation's most vulnerable populations (CMS, 2005). Six percent of Medicare beneficiaries account for 50 percent of Medicare spending. At least half of all funding for nursing home care is paid by the Medicaid program. Two groups of beneficiaries with extensive health care needs–those over age 85 and those with end stage renal disease (ESRD)–are the two fastest growing segments of the Medicare population. Medicare is an entitlement program for the aged and disabled. The disproportionate distribution of expenditures has influenced the adoption of practices and benefit eligibility that prioritize the identification of vulnerable or at risk individuals. This perspective is evident across a range of services and levels of care as reviewed below. It has also influenced attempts to create risk-adjusted payment levels for managed care enrollees, hospital inpatients, and the treatment/management of various chronic conditions.

Consumer Choice. A second cross cutting perspective influencing CMS practices is that of consumer choice. This is evident in data systems designed to provide consumers with information about the quality of care in hospitals and nursing homes, and in the opportunities given to beneficiaries to change providers and health plans.

Within Levels of Care. A third characteristic of CMS efforts is that many are oriented to performance monitoring and improving efficiencies *within* levels of care (e.g., hospitals, nursing homes, home care). Transitions between levels of care, or providers, or between financing systems are addressed in various ways. For example, some initiatives attempt to improve access to and the range of services offered at one level of care (e.g., primary care) with the hope of minimizing the need for more intensive and/or expensive care (often defined by hospital care). These approaches (e.g., disease management) may use interdisciplinary teams (e.g., physicians, nurses, social workers) in the treatment of vulnerable patients. Such interventions demonstrate awareness of the multi-dimensional needs of patients, but team involvement may be limited to specific settings (e.g., outpatient clinics, nursing homes), rather than carrying over to different levels of care or even the transitions between levels of care.

Case Management. The integration or transition between levels of care often relies on case management. There may be case managers at many points of transition across the continuum of care, but responsibility for any one is typically limited to the interface between two levels or settings of care. Case management takes many staffing forms, but with common elements. One of these is that of a gatekeeper who helps determine program or benefit eligibility. This function is common in access to long term care benefits, such as home care services and nursing homes, but it also applies to disease management or other approaches where the goal is to target program enrollment to specific levels of vulnerability. A variation on the gatekeeper role can be seen in hospitals where case managers (often called discharge planners) help expedite discharge from hospital. This can minimize hospital expenditures while shifting patient coverage to other providers.

A second function of case management is to improve communication (e.g., treatment plans, tests/laboratory results) between providers responsible for each of the interfacing levels of care. This is exemplified by the role of hospitalists in acute care; multidisciplinary teams involved with the transition from hospital to nursing home care; multidisciplinary teams that may be involved with complex patient needs among those in nursing homes, community settings or in advanced illness care; and social service support to physicians in addressing vulnerable populations in community settings. In almost all of these examples an implicit goal is to reduce preventable hospital stays/days and emergency room use. Rarely are there mechanisms for sharing cost savings between the interfacing delivery modalities.

A third case management function is to educate/inform/facilitate the "patient" or care recipient in fulfilling their responsibility in care or treatment compliance. Included here may be training in how to modify personal behaviors. An example of this function is the management of selected chronic diseases like diabetes and congestive heart failure. Another example is the broker role of helping the patient or care recipient gain access to benefits provided by another organization or another unit within the organization. Usually this is through a referral to these other programs (such as home care, or mental health services). The case manager in this role does not have responsibility over program eligibility or the level of assistance authorization.

A fourth function is that of quality assurance monitoring. Sometimes this is combined with supervising care providers. Commonly this is a periodic affirmation that the care provided is of adequate quality and quantity.

Financial Incentives. CMS continues to evaluate financial incentives as a means to affect provider behavior. This has taken a variety of forms. Among these are risk-adjusted capitation reimbursement for health plans and providers; and prospective payment for hospital stays, selected surgical procedures, and nursing home stays. These approaches are usually limited to specific levels or types of care, and a single source of payment such as Medicare or Medicaid. Disease management programs offer an example of a targeted payment and delivery model. The Social Health Maintenance Organizations, since transitioned into the regular managed care program, illustrate a more ambitious (and less specific) approach. These plans received extra payment to cover the expenses associated with an expansion of Medicare coverage to include social and other services not usually reimbursed under Medicare. Recipients of these services were usually persons with ADL limitations. The PACE program is CMS' most extensive attempt to combine Medicaid and Medicare into joint capitation financing. PACE is limited to those eligible for nursing home care, but the organization receives payment and assumes financial risk for all levels and duration of care depicted in Figure 1. Other integrative efforts include hospice care targeted at those near death, and EverCare which is a care coordination effort directed to persons in nursing homes.

The use of financial incentives may incorporate some aspect of risk sharing between the government and the provider. There have also been some directives such as the minimum types of benefits that must be covered, and constraints on service area, or enrollee eligibility. CMS has been less directive relative to operational structure, provider networks, and member recruitment/marketing, but such activities require prior approval. Evaluations of the financial incentive-related interventions and have typically focused on patient outcomes (like hospital and nursing home use, and expenditures relative to capitation payments), and enrollment and retention rates of both beneficiaries and providers. Relatively little study has been made of the specific organizational features developed within these innovative programs nor of the clinical practices that may have contributed to the program's performance.

Largely, but not completely missing among CMS financial initiatives projects are studies looking at alternative sources of revenue and the effects of these revenue sources on access to care and providers. Currently, this effort is limited to a study of the use of reverse mortgages as a potential means to finance portions of long term care expenses and another study examining asset transfers and the effect of this on eligibility for Medicaid. Studies of natural experiments, such as private long term care insurance in the U.S. or the implementation of public long term care insurance programs in other countries, are not priorities at the present. The effects of reimbursement on provider recruitment and retention are also not specific priorities, although elements of these issues are sometimes included in evaluations of state or other demonstrations. Concerns about tracking provider supply are largely within other federal agencies, such as the Health Resources and Services Administration (HRSA).

Population Health & Expenditures Across the Continuum of Care. The monitoring of population health and health care expenditures is distributed among a number of federal agencies and produce scores of surveys and data sources. Most of this work is conducted by units within the Department of Health & Human Services (DHHS), the department where CMS is located, but not by CMS itself. Data sources, among many others, include the National Health Interview Survey, a cross sectional survey of the community dwelling population; the Medical Expenditures Panel Survey (MEPS); and the National Long Term Care Survey (NLTCS). MEPS is a nationally representative survey. It includes a community dwelling household component and medical provider component. There is also a separate survey of nursing home residents. Household members are periodically resurveyed over 2 1/2 years to obtain information on medical use and expenditures. The NLTCS begins selecting a community sample, but tracks these individuals over time regardless of setting. Since 1982, this survey has linked to Medicare Part A & B claims data. It does not link to Medicaid.

Notable in reviewing the various data sources available through DHHS is that few have a sample size sufficient to monitor the experience (and service use/expenditures) of individuals across the continuum of care. Another limitation in the panel studies is that the samples do not generalize to individual states. The surveys and data systems sponsored by CMS generally have similar limitations. However, there is an infrastructure that could extend this work. One of these resources is the Medicare Current Beneficiary Survey (MCBS), a stratified national probability sample of aged and disabled beneficiaries, selected without regard to community or other dwelling location. This survey retains an individual in the panel for three years. CMS has also funded studies that compile service use and expenditures information on individuals across various settings or levels of care (e.g., hospital use by those in nursing homes). A full continuum of care data source is maintained by the PACE program.

EXPERIENCE WITH INTEGRATIVE CARE

This synopsis of CMS research and demonstration initiatives has highlighted approaches that address transitions between levels of care, and identified opportunities inherent within selected CMS programs that could be used to extend our knowledge about service use and their interactions along the continuum of care. This section provides a more detailed on several attempts to achieve care integration over some phases in the continuum of care.

Disease Management

Disease Management (DM) is a population-based approach to the outpatient treatment of several selected diseases (e.g., diabetes, congestive heart failure, chronic obstructive pulmonary disease). These programs are directed at individuals with a "high, but modifiable risk of adverse medical outcomes" (Foote, 2004: 342). Treatment is expected to follow normative interventions developed for each stage of the specific disease cycle. In addition to medical care, DM programs typically offer motivational/supportive services including telephone calls from program staff to encourage treatment (e.g., medications, diet, exercise) adherence; access to 24-hour nurse call centers; educational materials by mail, internet, or video, home health visits, biometric monitoring equipment (with or without calls that track vital statistics); and appointment or medical reminders. Many private-sector payers sponsor voluntary enrollment DM programs, and CMS has demonstrations testing DM in Medicare (Foote, 2004). The interest and adoption of DM is in part based on the intuitive appeal of the program, but early studies have shown efficacy and cost effectiveness (Weingarten et al., 2002). Another value of DM programs is that they build bridges between the often distinct domains of health education, medical care, and health monitoring. There is also an opportunity to bridge DM to long-term care. The common goal to maximize functioning and minimize intensive care needs suggest that the parallel programs of DM and personal and social care services may benefit by greater integration. Protocols for DM in a skilled nursing home population are being developed.

Other integrative interventions in out-patient care are group visit models and geriatric evaluation and management (GEM) programs. Two approaches to the group visit model have been replicated. The first targets patients with multiple chronic conditions, and the second addresses a specific chronic illness (e.g., diabetes) or grouping of conditions. Both approaches share similar program goals and features. To overcome discordance between the needs of those with chronic condition(s) and the typical primary care visit, group models strive to maximize the interaction between providers and patients by holding frequently scheduled (e.g., monthly) sessions with a multi-disciplinary provider team and approximately eight to twenty patients. The sessions emphasize education, self-management, and peer support. Many group programs also allow for individual patient visits with providers after the group sessions.

Measures of emergency department utilization, hospitalizations, patient satisfaction, and cost of care have demonstrated that group models may be able to overcome traditional barriers in the delivery system and reduce care fragmentation. Coleman and colleagues (2001) randomized control group trial of group visits for elder patients with multiple chronic conditions demonstrated a reduced rate of emergency department visits (0.65 versus 1.08 during a 2 year follow-up). Similarly, Wagner, Grothaus, and colleagues' (2001) randomized control trial at a diabetes clinic in Seattle, Washington found that patients assigned to intervention groups received more preventative procedures and had fewer specialty and emergency room visits.

GEM programs are an outgrowth of the Comprehensive Geriatric Assessment (CGA), a model that was introduced in the late 1980s, that emphasizes interdisciplinary assessment of an older person's medical, functional, and psychosocial status, in order to develop a comprehensive treatment plan (Reuben, 2002). Early studies of CGA found that interdisciplinary assessment was not enough to affect elder patient hospital utilization and that costs associated with in-patient CGA were high. These issues stimulated an extension of the CGA model that included treatment and on-going patient management in out-patient settings. Many of the early trials of out-patient GEM programs identified positive results on measures of patient satisfaction, quality of health and social care, and hospital utilization, but were not able to demonstrate improved health and functional status. More targeted GEM programs have been able to demonstrate some improvements in functional status. Boult et al.'s (2001) investigation of functional ability and use and cost of health care services among high risk community-based elders in Minnesota identified a slowed functional decline for those randomized into a GEM intervention group. However, cost of care outcomes were less conclusive. In most cases (75%), no relationship between group assignment and total care expenditures was identified. In the remaining 25% of cases, cost for the GEM group was higher. Although the initial investment required to provide GEM care may be more expensive than standard care, over time this investment may be realized for its ability to decrease in-patient or institutional care costs. Unfortunately, trials periods may be too short for a measurable return on investment to be seen.

Despite some gaps in our knowledge of DM, group practice and GEM programs, these interventions have been successful in stimulating a re-conceptualization of primary care practice reflective of more effective chronic care management protocols. Policy has set the environment for the development of local initiatives, and in turn, these initiatives inform policy. The relationship or feedback loop between local experience and policy is one that should be continually encouraged and supported so that the health care environment continually stimulates and supports the development of creative programs, and creative programs can continue to test and improve upon existing deliver mechanisms that shape policy.

Inpatient Integration Interventions

The financial incentives on hospitals to shorten the length of stay and minimize readmissions have helped stimulate a number of efforts to improve inpatient care and to better link inpatient with post-acute care, including nursing homes. ACE units (Acute Care of the Elderly) are one example. The ACE unit concept was first described in the mid to late 1980s as a way of minimizing the functional decline experienced by elders following hospitalization due to processes of iatrogenesis, polypharmacy, immobilization and depersonalization (Covinsky et al., 1998). ACE units are targeted to elder subpopulations and may be offered in specially designed sections of hospitals or, more recently, as hospital-wide interventions. Included protocols are a multi-dimensional assessment linked to treatment aimed at maintaining neurocognitive and psychosocial function, medical care review to prevent iatrogenic complications, interdisciplinary team rounds, and home discharge planning (Reuben, 2002).

A randomized controlled trial at University Hospitals of Cleveland compared ACE unit care with usual in-patient care. Twenty-one percent of ACE patients reported a "much better" change in their ADL function between hospital admission and discharge compared to 13% of usual care patients (Covinsky et al., 1998). Higher daily costs associated with ACE unit care were balanced by a shorter average length of stay.

ACE unit protocols have also been developed for sleep enhancement, dehydration and feeding assistance, therapeutic activities, and sensory impairment adaptations. Saint Louis University Hospital has developed a Delirium Room (DR) program within their ACE unit and several hospitals including Summa Health System (SHS) Hospitals in Akron, Ohio, have used the ACE model rather than the traditional biomedical model for developing their stroke units (SU).

Despite a number of studies that demonstrate beneficial health, function, and potential for cost reduction, a 2003 survey identified that only 16 hospitals reported having introduced ACE units (Jayadevappa, Bloom, Raziano, & Livizzo-Mourey, 2003). Improved functional status and reduced nursing home use may not sufficiently reduce the cost per case for hospitals nor provide the incentive to change organizational or administrative structures to implement ACE units. Aligning demonstrated effective programs with policy that stimulates their replication is an important challenge that must be met. Reimbursement incentives that motivate hospitals to develop programs such as ACE units may be one approach to addressing the quality and cost tradeoffs that influence the organization of care and treatment decisions for higher need patients.

Other approaches to bridge the domains of primary, hospital, and sub-acute care have been developed for nursing home patients. One variation uses primary care physicians (often teamed with a nurse practitioner) to manage inpatient care and to conduct frequent patient visits. An augmentation on this uses a multi-disciplinary team that practices exclusively with nursing home, home care and hospice patients. CMS has financed a capitation version of this model called EverCare. The intensive patient monitoring and collaboration between the primary care physician/nurse practitioner and the nursing home are expected to minimize hospitalizations.

Findings from these interventions were favorable. The primary care/ nurse practitioner model showed similar health care utilization levels as fee-for service patients, but lower overall costs of care (Reuben, 2002). The dedicated team approach resulted in fewer transfers to the Emergency Department and had a smaller percentage of residents hospitalized compared with fee-for-service residents (Kane, Flood, Bershadsky, & Keckhafer, 2004). Both programs improved processes of care (i.e., provider response times to patient issues).

PACE Model of Integrated Care

PACE is the one service program that has integrated financing across the full continuum of care. PACE is jointly funded by Medicare and Medicaid using capitated payment. Enrollment in the managed care program is targeted to non-institutionalized persons age 55 and over who meet the frailty criteria. The PACE program began in 1972. It was eventually replicated in 15 locations before amendments to Medicare and Medicaid allowed PACE as a Medicare benefit and provider type in 1997 (Titles XVII and XIX of the Social Security Act as part of the Balanced Budget Act of 1997). Today, the PACE model of care is offered at 32 sites in 22 states and serves approximately 13,000 frail elder enrollees. Another 11 sites are operating with Medicare capitation while state Medicaid waiver applications are pending.

Service Integration. PACE provides or finances most of the services in the continuum of care shown in Figure 1. These include hospital, nursing home, and specialty care which are contracted, as well as primary care and a range of non-medical services. Primary care and non-medical services are provided by PACE employees. Each PACE site uses an interdisciplinary team for primary care/care management across all levels of care. These teams include primary care physicians, nurse practitioners, clinical nurses, home health nurses, social workers, occupational and physical therapists, dietitians, health workers, recreation therapists, and transportation workers (Eng, Pedulla, Eleazer, McCann, & Fox, 1997). PACE has discretion in allocating resources among its array of primary, acute care, supportive and social care, home care, palliative care, and nursing home care (Johri, Beland, & Bergman, 2003). PACE sites also operate or have alliances with low income housing programs. These are not funded under the PACE payment, but many enrollees reside and receive PACE assistance in this housing.

In addition to the provider "lock-in" features, PACE has one more striking feature. Enrollees are encouraged to regularly attend the program's adult day health center (attendance three days per week is the average) (National PACE Association). The day centers provide full-service medical clinic care, and all facilities necessary for social and rehabilitation services.

Unlike case management as a facilitator of level of care transitioning in other CMS delivery systems, PACE links the provision of services and the management of care to the same multi-disciplinary team (Johri, et al., 2003). This consolidation is thought to promote cross-reporting and communication between team members throughout the cycles of care: assessment, treatment plans, service allocation and delivery, treatment monitoring, and care plan adjustment.

PACE providers operate at full financial risk for all costs associated medical, hospital, and nursing home care. PACE providers have no opportunity to shift costs from one payer to another. Instead they have the means to "recover" savings from higher cost care, if they are able to deliver an appropriate array of less expensive services (Eng et al., 1997).

PACE Evaluations. In spite of its uniqueness, most studies of PACE have been conducted to measure performance and assure that the capitation formulas were equitable to the government, rather to gain insight into the effectiveness of particular clinical practices. This is beginning to change. Studies of hospital stays and skilled nursing home utilization have shown PACE members to have use rates below those of comparably frail Medicare managed care or fee-for service populations (Tempkin-Greener & Mukamel, 2002; Wieland et al., 2000). Hospitalization per annum was 2,158 days per 1000 patients per year among PACE members. This compares to 2,080 days per 1000 patients per year among Medicare beneficiaries who on average had fewer ADL dependencies than PACE enrollees who average 4 ADL limitations at time of enrollment (Wieland et al., 2000). Further, hospitals as the location of death was lower for PACE enrollees (21%) compared to the 65+ general population who die in hospital (50%) (Tempkin-Greener & Mukamel, 2002), and length of hospital stay was shorter for PACE enrollees compared to an older Medicare population (4.8 vs. 6.0 days) (Eng et al., 1997).

Another area of concern for CMS has been how PACE Medicare and Medicaid capitation payments compare to the cost of serving frail elders in a fee-for service environment (Robinson & Karon, 2000). Comparisons are complicated by the difficulty of obtaining a "comparable group," but the available data show that PACE produces savings for Medicare ranging from 12% to 39% (Eng et al., 1997). These studies will likely be replicated as PACE begins implementing a new risk-adjusted payment methodology introduced in 2004. Medicaid capitation payments are negotiated separately in each state, but follow a common framework. Internal studies comparing PACE performance with fee for service beneficiaries identified as certified eligible for nursing home care yield an estimated 5% to 15% savings among PACE enrollees (Eng et al., 1997).

CMS has been slow to launch studies and demonstrations that explore specific elements of the PACE model of care. Two exceptions are the Wisconsin Partnership Program (WPP) and the Minnesota Senior Health Options/Minnesota Disability Health Options (MSHO) programs. The WPP was developed as a collaborative approach to integrating health and long-term care that linked the resources of existing provider organizations. Under a Medicaid Section 1115/ Medicare Section 222 waiver, the state was given authority to develop a PACE-like program that would offer more choice in primary care providers and relax the day center focus of PACE (Ryan & Super, 2003). Like PACE, the majority of participants at WPP are dually-eligible, community-dwelling, nursing home certifiable elders. However, a small percent of WPP participants are disabled individuals between the age of 18 and 64 years.

The WPP is operational at four sites. Two sites, Community Care for the Elderly in Milwaukee and ElderCare in Madison, originally ran both WPP and PACE programs concurrently. However, after two years, ElderCare merged the two programs, selecting the Partnership model (Gross, Tempkin-Greener, Kunitz, & Mukamel, 2004). The third site, Community Living Alliance, in Madison serves individuals aged 18-64 with physical disabilities. The fourth site, Community Health Partnership in Eau Claire, serves both disabled and elder populations (Wisconsin Department of Health and Family Services (DHFS), 2000).

Addressing consumer concerns about having to give up their primary care physicians upon enrolling in PACE, the WPP allows participants to select their physician from an independent physician panel, or continue with their existing primary care provider. Also differing from the PACE model, the Partnership program does not require direct participation of the primary care physician in team meetings. Nurse practitioners assume responsibility for coordinating the teams' activities with community-based physicians and may even accompany enrollees to office visits with the physician (Ryan & Super, 2003). An additional difference between WPP and PACE is a reduced reliance on day centers as a structure to provide services. WPP is primarily a home-based program (Wisconsin DHFS, 2000).

Early findings of the WPP suggest that non-staff physicians may not be able to address client needs as well as staff physicians and that the absence of a staff physician also increased burden on other interdisciplinary team members (Kane, Homyak, Bershadsky, & Lum, 2002). However, enrollee outcomes data suggests positive results on measures of self-determination and choice, community integration, and health and safety, and positive impact on the rate of hospital admissions for conditions of diabetes, congestive heart failure, pneumonia, and chronic obstructive pulmonary disease (Wisconsin DHFS, 2001).

Like PACE, the MSHO program is a managed care program that pools Medicare and Medicaid funding to create a more integrated acute, primary and long-term care delivery system for Minnesota's dually eligible population. Unlike PACE, the MSHO program serves individuals living in either community or in institutional settings and does not require individuals to be nursing home certifiable to qualify for enrollment.

The MSHO program was introduced as a demonstration program in 1997 in seven counties around the Minneapolis and St. Paul metropolitan areas. The program was designed as a means to align financial incentives with best practices, reduce service delivery fragmentation, and reduce cost shifting between the Medicare and Medicaid. The MSHO program is a voluntary option to the standard Prepaid Medical Assistance Program (PMAP) program in which most Medicaid eligible seniors in Minnesota are required to enroll. Those that do not enroll continue to receive Medicare-covered services through fee-for-service and PMAP Medicaid services.

The Minnesota Department for Human Services (DHS) which runs the MSHO program obtained federal waivers to select three contractors (Medica, UCare, and Metropolitan Health) to provide a full range of integrated services on a capitated risk basis (National Chronic Care Consortium, 2001). These health plans in turn subcontract with a number of health systems and providers to offer a full compliment of services (Kane, Homyak, Bershadsky, Flood, & Zhang, 2004). In order to coordinate services and providers, care coordinators are assigned to every program enrollee. As DHS did not dictate any one model, several care coordination models are being used simultaneously. Some use geriatric nurse practitioners who work exclusively in nursing home settings, other care coordination models use social workers or registered nurses who work out of clinics or community settings. The use of separate care coordination models allows for greater provider flexibility, but may also lead to confusion and duplication.

Although early outcomes of the MSHO program found only modest advantages (Kane, Weiner, Homyak, & Bershadsky, 2001; Kane, Homyak, Bershadsky, Lum, & Said Siadaty, 2003), a more recent quasi-experimental control group study demonstrated more favorable results, particularly for MSHO nursing home enrollees. On eight measures of hospital utilization and professional encounters, Kane et al. (2004) identified that the community dwelling MSHO intervention group had fewer preventable hospital admissions (.71 versus .92 average monthly per 100) and fewer face to face physician visits (79.5 versus 121.6 average monthly per 100) compared to the control group after 18 months. The MSHO nursing home intervention group had significantly lower hospitalization and professional encounters on all eight measures. More than previous studies, Kane et al. (2004) identified that a dual-eligible targeted program can reduce medical service utilization. However, like PACE, further investigation of which components of the MSHO program have contributed to these results is required. EverCare, a major contractor for MSHO nursing home care has demonstrated effective results as a managed care provider. Thus, the effects of other program components such as pooled Medicare and Medicaid funding require further study (Kane et al., 2004).

Other studies underway that explore elements of the PACE model include palliation and end of life care (Ryan, Tuuk, & Lee, 2004; Mukamel, Bajorska, & Tempkin-Greener, 2002), and the impact of clinical protocols (e.g., rate of hip fractures) (Walter, Lui, Eng, & Covinsky, 2003).

DISCUSSION

The Continuum of Care

The research and demonstration programs sponsored by CMS address all the dimensions of the continuum of care. This is accomplished in a piecemeal fashion, but there are common perspectives that likely will continue to be reflected in program and policy design going forward. Key among these are emphases supporting consumer choice, and the paradox of favoring capitation payment as a means to encourage utilization control and to influence provider behavior, and a targeting of benefits and integrative strategies to relatively easily identified vulnerable populations.

Another attribute of CMS efforts is a focus on efficiency/performance within a single level of care or service setting. Other than programs directed to the interface between two levels of care, few initiatives encompass multiple phases in the continuum of care. There have been examples of risk sharing, but partnerships between CMS and the providers/states directed toward the development of interventions tend to be relatively short term (e.g., 3-5) years. This allows little time for the provider organizations to establish and refine their procedures and practices–this may reduce the likelihood of obtaining the hoped for effectiveness. Ideas, such as case management, have been able to survive negative evaluation findings and have expanded into general practice, but other ideas may have faltered during their early development phases.

The PACE Program

Recognition of where we are in the development and testing of policy and practices across the continuum of care is a helpful. It can serve as a starting point for reassessing the approaches taken and in prioritizing the gaps in knowledge yet to be addressed. Disease management, long term care financing, and further refinement of risk adjusted payment methodologies are issues with on-going importance and priority, and likely have a momentum that will extend work in these areas. To this list of priorities, we suggest adding a planned research program directed at the one CMS program, PACE, that spans the full continuum of care.

This suggestion reflects a desire (1) to better understand the interaction of practices and their consequences across the continuum of care that can be observed within PACE, and (2) to gain insight into practices that might be transferable to traditional managed care or fee for service systems. Relatively little is known about the efficacy of specific clinical practices within PACE, and whether all features (e.g., staff physicians, adult day care attendance, constant interdisciplinary teams across all levels of care) must be present for cost effective performance. Would PACE enrollment grow if consumers had more discretion in selecting their physicians, hospitals, and nursing homes; and/or if they were given more discretion about whether or how frequently they attended day care programs? How would such changes affect health care use, expenditures, and member outcomes? Can the historic PACE efficiencies and performance be maintained if member eligibility were broadened beyond those defined as nursing home certifiable, such as targeted diseases, and/or those with terminal illness?

CMS, at the initiative of states and providers, has begun to test some versions of the PACE model in two states. Can the process of innovation and refinement in the delivery system be accelerated? PACE programs already have comprehensive health and long term care coverage and financing. Is it possible for CMS, the states, and PACE providers to collaboratively develop strategic plan for testing innovations? Under such a model, PACE sites, in addition to their on-going operations, would be asked to function as "laboratories" to develop and test new approaches. Some of this work might include efficacy studies unbundling selected traditional internal practices. Other work would test the effects of variations in practice. Efficacious work might eventually be extended to other settings and providers. Such a collaborative approach between CMS, the states, and PACE could lead to the development of a more structured feedback system between local organizations and policy that could enhance our learning of demonstrations and accelerate practice and policy refinements.

CONCLUSION

In conclusion, while the development of policy and research activity relative to the continuum of care has often been piecemeal, many elements are in place. Programs emphasizing consumer choice, pooled Medicare and Medicaid funding, and integrative delivery strategies have begun to change health and long-term care delivery for vulnerable populations. Support for and knowledge of programs directed at multiple phases of the care continuum have the potential to produce even greater change. Strategic use of Centers of Excellence resources like the community-based PACE program offer much potential for extending and refining knowledge and practice into how to implement care integration and thereby effectively influence social policy.

REFERENCES

Boult, C., Boult, L. B., Morishita, L., Dowd, B., Kane, R. L., & Urdangarin, C. F. (2001). A randomized clinical trial of outpatient geriatric evaluation and management. *Journal of the American Geriatrics Society*, 49(4), 351-359.

Cassel, Besdine, & Siegel, 1999 Restructuring Medicare for the next century: What will beneficiaries really need? *Health Affairs*, 18(1), 118-131.

Centers for Medicare & Medicaid Services (CMS). (2005) *CMS Research Activities: The Active Projects Report.* http://www.cms.hhs.gov/researchers/projects/apr/default.asp.

Coleman, E. A., Eilertsen, T. B., Kramer, A. M., Magid, D. J., Beck, A., & Conner, D. (2001). Reducing emergency visits in older adults with chronic illness. A randomized, controlled trial of group visits. *Effective Clinical Practice*, 4(2), 49-57.

Covinsky, K. E., Palmer, R. M., Kresevic, D. M., Kahana, E., Counsell, S. R., Fortinsky, R. H. et al. (1998). Improving functional outcomes in older patients: Lessons from an acute care for the elderly unit. *Journal on Quality Improvement*, 24(2), 63-76.

Eng, C., Pedulla, J., Eleazer, P., McCann, R., & Fox, N. (1997). Program of All-Inclusive Care for the Elderly: An innovative model of integrated geriatric care and financing. *Journal of the American Geriatrics Society*, 45(2), 223-232.

Gross, D. L., Tempkin-Greener, H., Kunitz, S., & Mukamel, D. B. (2004). The growing pains of integrated health care for the elderly: Lessons from the expansion of PACE. *The Milbank Quarterly*, 82(2), 257-282.

Jayadevappa, R., Bloom, B. S., Raziano, D. B., & Lavizzo-Mourey, R. (2003). Dissemination and characteristics of acute care for elders (ACE) units in the United States. *International Journal of Technology Assessment in Health Care*, 19(1), 220-227.

Johri, M., Beland, F., & Bergman, H. (2003). International experiments in integrated care for the elderly: A synthesis of the evidence. *International Journal of Geriatric Psychiatry*, 18, 222-235.

Kane, R. L., Flood, S., Bershadsky, B., & Keckhafer, G. (2004). Effect of an innovative Medicare managed care program on the quality of nursing home residents. *The Gerontologist*, 44(1), 95-103.

Kane, R. L., Homyak, P., & Bershadsky, B. (2002). Consumer reactions to the Wisconsin Partnership Program and its parent, the Program for All-Inclusive Care of the Elderly. *The Gerontologist*, 42(3), 314-320.

Kane, R. L., Homyak, P., Bershadsky, B., Flood, S., & Zhang, H. (2004). Patterns of utilization for the Minnesota Senior Health Options Program. *Journal of the American Geriatrics Society*, 52(12), 2039-2044.

Kane, R. L., Homyak, P., Bershadsky, B., & Lum, Y. S. (2002). Consumer responses to the Wisconsin Partnership Program for elderly persons: A variation on the PACE model. *Journal of Gerontology*, 57(4), M250-258.

Kane, R. L., Homyak, P., & Bershadsky, B., Lum, Y. S., & Said Siadaty, M. (2003). Outcomes of managed care of dually eligible older persons. *The Gerontologist*, 43(2), 165-174.

Kane, R. L., Weiner, A., Homyak, P., & Bershadsky, B. (2001). The Minnesota Senior Health Options Program: An early effort at integrating care for the dually-eligible. *Journal of Gerontology: Medical Sciences*, 56A(9), M559-M566.

Mukamel, D. B., Bajorska, A., & Tempkin-Greener, H. (2002). Health care services utilization at the end of life in a managed care program integrating acute and long-term care. *Medical Care,* 40(12), 1136-1148.

National Chronic Care Consortium. (2001, March). Provider survey report: Summary of 2000 survey of MSHO care coordinators, nurse practitioners, and physicians. Retrieved April 27, 2005, from http://www.ncconline.org/products/M09001.pdf

National PACE Association. (n.d.). Frequently asked questions about PACE. Retrieved March 1, 2005 from http://www.npaonline.org/website/article.asp?id=24/

Reuben, D. B. (2002). Organizational interventions to improve health outcomes of older persons. *Medical Care,* 40(5), 416-428.

Robinson, J. & Karon, S. L. (2000). Modeling Medicare costs of PACE populations. *Health Care Financing Review*, 21(3), 149-170.

Ryan, J. & Super, N. (2003, September). *Dually eligible for Medicare and Medicaid: Two for one or double jeopardy?* (National Health Policy Forum Issue Brief No. 794). Washington, DC: George Washington University.

Ryan, S. D., Tuuk, M., & Lee, M. (2004). PACE and hospice: Two models on the verge of collaboration. *Clinical Geriatric Medicine*, 20(4), 783-794.

Stone, R. I. & Katz, R. (1996). Thoughts on the future of integrating acute and long-term care. In R. Newcomer and A. Wilkersin (Eds.), *Annual review of gerontology and geriatrics*, Volume 16. New York, NY: Springer.

Tempkin-Greener, H. & Mukamel, D. B. (2002). Predicting place of death in the program of All-inclusive Care for the Elderly (PACE): Participant versus program characteristics. *Journal of the American Geriatric Society*, 50(1), 125-135.

Villagra, V. G. (2004). Integrating disease management into the outpatient delivery system during and after managed care [Electronic version]. *Health Affairs*, (W4), 281-283.

Wagner, E. H., Austin, B., Davis, C., Hindmarsh, M., Schaefer, J., & Bonomi, A. (2001). Improving chronic illness care: Translating evidence into action. *Health Affairs*, 20(6), 64-78.

Wagner, E. H., Grothaus, L. C., Sandhu, N., Galvin, M. S., McGregor, M., Artz, K. et al. (2001). Chronic care clinics for Diabetes in primary care. *Diabetes Care*, 25(4), 695-700.

Walter, L. C., Lui, L. Y., Eng, C., & Covinsky, K. E. (2003). Risk of hip fracture in disabled community-living older adults. *Journal of the American Geriatrics Society*, 51(1), 50-55.

Weingarten, S. R., Henning, J. M., Badamgarav, E., Knight, K., Hasselbald, V., Gano, A. et al. (2002). Interventions used in disease management programmes for patients with chronic illness–which ones work? Meta-analysis of published reports. *British Medical Journal*, 325, 925-928.

Whitelaw, N. A. & Warden, G. L. (1999). Reexamining the delivery system as a part of Medicare reform. *Health Affairs*, 18(1), 132-143.

Wieland, D., Lamb, V. L., Sutton, S. R., Boland, R., Clark, M., Friedman, S. et al. (2000). Hospitalization in the Program of All-Inclusive Care for the elderly (PACE): Rates, concomitants, and predictors. *Journal of the American Geriatrics Society*, 48(11), 1373-1380.

Wiener, J. M. & Stevenson, D. G. (1998). State policy on long-term care for the elderly. *Health Affairs*, 17(3), 81-100.

Wisconsin Department of Health and Family Services (2000, September). Wisconsin Partnership Program: An integrated care model. Retrieved May 4, 2005, from http://dhfs.wisconsin.gov

Wisconsin Department of Health and Family Services. (2001, July). Partnership quality. Member outcomes: An initial assessment. Retrieved May 2, 2005, from http://dhfs.state.wi.us/Wipartnership/pdf-wpp/Member%20Partnership070901FINAL.pdf

When the Private Sphere Goes Public: Exploring the Issues Facing Family Caregiver Organizations in the Development of Long-Term Care Policies

Philip A. Rozario
Elizabeth Palley

INTRODUCTION

Families have long helped meet the caregiving needs of their frail, dependent and disabled members. Indeed, many argue that the family is the backbone of the American long-term care system, providing much of the required services to frail relatives and absorbing much of the caregiving-related costs (Stone, Cafferata, & Sangl, 1987; Walker, 1983). The family's importance in the long-term care system is reflected in their efforts to maintain the frail relative in the community, thus delaying or preventing institutional care.

From a demographic viewpoint, long-term caregiving to frail older adults is a fairly recent phenomenon. The dramatic increase in life expectancy in the U.S., from 47 years in 1900 to approximately 76 years currently, and the advances in medical technology that allow more people to live with chronic health conditions have contributed to this phenomenon (Feinberg et al., 2003). The National Alliance for Caregiving (NAC) and the AARP (2004) estimate that 21% of the U.S. population are caregivers to friends and relatives ages 18 and older, numbering more than 44 million caregivers. Thus, families are often faced with the question of how to provide for their dependent elders on a long-term basis. Further, women, who tend to be the primary family caregivers, can expect to spend more time looking after their parents than their children (Bengtson, Giarusson, Silverstein, & Wang, 2000).

In this paper, we address some of the long-term care policy issues as they pertain to caregivers of older adults. In the next section, we review the definition of caregiving and the tasks caregivers perform in meeting the needs of their frail older relatives. We explore the divide between the public and private spheres and then, provide an overview of family caregiving-related policies and programs in the U.S. In our review, we examine the provisions in the NFCSP, Medicaid waiver legislation, and

Family and Medical Leave Act that support of family caregiving efforts as well as their provisions for advocacy by and on behalf family caregivers. Finally, we assess the roles of family caregiver organizations in making family caregiving an important element of long-term care policy, especially in highlighting the challenges that they face, their successes, and also their future in influencing policy-making.

What Is Caregiving?

Caregiving usually refers to the in-kind services that people provide to other functionally dependent people. These in-kind services have been categorized as assistance with instrumental activities of daily living (IADL), which refer to activities that are important in managing one's daily life or maintaining one's household; and assistance with activities of daily living (ADL), which refer to activities that involve personal care (NAC & AARP, 1997). Like most of the services within the long-term care system, informal caregiving services straddle the fields of health, personal and social services that are provided to people "who have lost or never acquired some degree of functional capacity" (Kane & Kane, 1987, p. 4).

The performances of IADL and ADL tasks are related, to some extent, to the care receivers' functioning and cognitive abilities. Using the 1982 National Long-term Care Survey, Stone, Cafferata, and Sangl (1982) found that 67.2% of the caregivers in their sample reported performing hygiene-related personal care, 45.7% reported helping with mobility, and 80.6% reported performing household chores. More recently, the NAC and AARP (2004) found that 80% of their sample provided IADL assistance in three or more IADL areas, and 26% reported providing ADL assistance in three or more ADL areas.

The number of caregiving hours increases with the level of functional impairments experienced by the care receivers. Stone, Cafferata, and Sangl (1987) found that, on the average, caregivers provide up to four hours of care daily. The NAC and AARP (2004) survey found that one-fifth of their sample provided 40 hours or more per week. They also found that in comparison to caregivers who provided less care, those who provided more than 40 hours of care were likely to live with their care receiver, be over 65 years of age, and have lower income and lower levels of educational attainment. In separate analyses of National Long-Term Care Survey data, White-Means and Thornton (1990) found that black caregivers were likely to spend 9 to 12 hours more providing care than their white counterparts.

Despite researchers' and clinicians' focus on the help that caregivers provide in meeting the ADL and IADL needs of their care receivers, caregivers often end up doing more than just meeting the activities for daily living needs of their dependent relatives. Indeed the measurement of the ADL and IADL assistance provided by caregivers do not completely reflect the complexity of the demands caregivers face in meeting their care receivers' needs. Carol Levine and her colleagues argue that caregivers, for the most part, give selflessly of themselves, and do whatever needs to be done to ensure the comfort and well-being of their older relatives in the face of declining health and physical functioning (Levine & Hart, 2004). Though a better measure of the efforts of caregivers would be one that includes the timing of care, the proximity required of caregivers in the tasks they do, the level of their caregiving efforts, and how active care receivers are active in their care, the current measures demonstrate the high level of services that are currently being performed by family caregivers (Albert, 2004).

The Private versus the Public Spheres

Caregiving, like other family-related functions, has long been considered a phenomenon that occurs in the private realms of the family beyond the reaches of government and market influences (McGovern & Matter, 1992). Some researchers argue against this private-public dichotomy in asserting that "caregiving lies at the intersection of family, work, and government sectors and these three institutions mutually interact to shape caregiving experiences" (Silverstein & Parrott, 2001, p. 357). Indeed, the permeability of the private and public spheres is evident when we examine the spillover effects of work stress on the family life, and that of family stress on the work life. In a sample of 1,247 caregivers, the NAC and AARP (2004) found that 48% of the sample reported full time employment, while another 11% reported part-time employment. Working family caregivers are often faced with difficult decisions about prioritizing the demands of caregiving and work. Though only a small percentage of employed caregivers gave up their employment altogether, 57% reported that they went to work late, left early or took time off in order to provide care for their frail relatives (NAC & AARP, 2004).

Additionally, the public sphere has also affected the ability of family caregivers to provide care. For example, cost containment policies adopted by Medicare in the 1980s, beginning with the introduction of the Prospective Payment System, have led to a phenomenon where older people are being discharged from hospitals "quicker and sicker," leaving many family caregivers with demands that may include the management of medical-related equipment in addition to the physical assistance of grooming, bathing and help with toilet use. It is likely that the spiraling medical cost and cost containment efforts may continue to shift more of this burden to family caregivers.

Silverstein and Parrott (2001) argue that "the current political environment favors less government intrusion into the lives of individuals" (p. 353). In other words, the current climate does not favor supportive policies for family caregivers. Policies that deal with long-term care often fail to recognize the role of family caregivers or are likely to assume that family caregivers will provide care regardless of their availability or ability. Current long-term care policies lack coherence and do not provide a comprehensive approach to dealing with family caregivers. Additionally, according to Linsk, Keigher, Simon-Rusinowitz, and England (1992), policymakers may be hesitant to develop policies that are supportive of family caregiving for fear that the establishment of publicly-funded services would create woodwork and substitution effects. The fear being that the supply of services would create increased need among families and if formal care options were made available families would be more likely to substitute their informal care with formal care respectively.

POLICIES ON FAMILY CAREGIVING

The long-term care policies in the U.S. began in the 19th century with the focus on how best to deal with poverty and dependence among the population (OECD, 1996). Historically, long-term care policy has been tied to institutional care, beginning with the Elizabethean law, when institutionalization was seen as the as the best means to deal with the problems of care for the destitute elderly (OECD, 1996). The focus on institutional care remains to this day. Even though more frail elders are living in the community, nursing home care expenditure increased from $17.7 billion in 1980 to $110.8 billion in 2003 (Center for Medicare and Medicaid Services, 2005). The renewed focus on family caregiving can in part be attributed to the concern that long-term care services consume a major share of the total health care spending. Indeed, cost effectiveness of the U.S. long-term care policies depends on the continued reliance on family caregivers. After all, we can argue that family caregivers allow others to participate as in the civic, economic, and political life of society (Herd & Meyer, 2002). Hence, we need to consider the ways in which policies shape the caregiving experience and in turn, how caregivers can shape the policies that may affect their caregiving experiences.

In this section, we will review a number of long-term care policies that are specifically focused on family caregivers. Several pieces of recent federal legislation provided support for family caregiving including the Family and Medical Leave Act (FMLA, 1993), the National Family Caregiving Support Program (NFCSP), and the Medicaid Waiver programs.

The Family and Medical Leave Act

The Family and Medical Leave Act (FMLA) was passed in 1993 in an effort to ensure that, on a temporary basis, up to 12 weeks a year, employees were not fired for performing caregiving activities for their sick relatives, specifically, children, spouses, and/or parents. The law states that women are more often responsible for caregiving than men and are often forced to balance this responsibility while participating in the workforce. As a result, it was passed in order to ensure that women are not discriminated against in employment situations on the basis of their gender, that they receive equal protection and so that they are better able to balance their family and work responsibilities. Men, who chose to participate in caregiving responsibilities, are also covered under this law. In addition to allowing employees to take a leave for health reasons or the birth or adoption of a child, FMLA entitles employees to, "take reasonable leave for," caregiving activities associated with "a spouse, or parent who has a serious health condition" (PL 101-3, Section 2, Part B(2), 1993).

The FMLA represents the first major federal legislation that provides employed caregivers protected leave without pay for their caregiving responsibilities (Glass & Estes, 1997; Johnson & Sasso, 2000). The law applies only to employees who work in businesses that employ at least 50 people and who have worked for at least 1,250 hours in the past year (Department of Labor, 1993). This excludes 40% of the workforce (Wisensale, 2003). Though covered employers are required to continue to provide their employees on leave with benefits that are provided to other employees including, "group life insurance, health insurance, disability insurance, sick leave, annual leave, educational benefits, and pensions," (PL 103-3, Title I Section 101(5), 1993), they are not required to provide their employees with a salary during the leave. For many employed caregivers, this limits their ability to exercise their right to take a leave. Further, the FMLA allows eligible employers to deny

certain personnel, the highest paid ten percent of their employees to receive this benefit if the employer notifies the employees prior to their
leave and if "such denial is necessary to prevent substantial and griev-
ous economic injury to the operations of the employer" (PL 103-3, Title
I, Section 104(b), 1993). Lastly, the FMLA does not apply to care for an
extended family member, such as an adult sibling, an in-law, or to partners in a committed relationship (Wisensale, 2003).

In studying the implementation of the FMLA, Lechner and Neal
(1999) reported that employers were likely to create barriers to em-
ployee utilization of this benefit. In their study of 980 Californian firms,
they found that 40% of these firms were out of compliance with at least
one of the required provisions, such as posting notices, preparing leave
requesting forms, and training supervisors to be more sensitive. The
Commission on Family and Medical Leave and the Women's Bureau
(1996) reported that 86.5% of employers in FMLA-covered worksites
knew that the Act applied to their worksites and only 58.2% of their employees were aware of the FMLA. Further, they found that salaried
(versus hourly-waged), unionized (versus non-unionized), and higher
educated (versus less educated) workers were more aware of the provisions of the FMLA. Given the limitations of this law as well as the dis-
juncture between its goals and the implementation, in many instances, it
may be considered more symbolic than actually supportive of family
caregiving.

National Family Caregiver Support Program

The NFCSP (2000) was the first piece of federal legislation to provide
funding specifically for family caregiving support services (Feinberg &
Newman, 2004; Fox-Grave, Coleman, & Blancato, 2001). It is a grant
program to states that encourages, "multifaceted systems of support services... for family caregivers; and ... for grandparents or older individuals who are relative caregivers," (Subpart 1 Section 373, 2000).
These services may include access to information about services, assistance in obtaining services, counseling, support groups, respite
care, and "supplemental services, on a limited basis to complement the
care provided by caregivers" (Section 373(b), 2000). In other words, they
may support potentially any program that a state or area office on aging
develops to help facilitate family caregiving activities. The National
Association of State Units on Aging (NASUA) proposed a systemic
program development approach that is aimed at creating state-level
programs that are "accessible, flexible, consumer-directed, culturally

competent, and integrated with home and community-based services" (2003, p. 2).

A number of programs have been implemented to meet the needs of family caregivers of older adults in various states. According to the Administration on Aging (2004), these programs include the development of single-point-of-entry services and the adoption of family-directed service options. The NASUA (2003) highlighted the program in Maine where the Area Agencies on Aging have a single toll-free number that directs caregivers to the appropriate Area Agency. While consumer direction is inherent in the Older Americans' Act (Administration on Aging, 2003), North Dakota offers its caregivers a consumer-directed respite program where caregivers are given $1,900 per year to choose their respite service providers (NASUA, 2003). Further, in recognition of the discrepancy between the high need and low service utilization by ethnic minority elders and their families, NASUA (2003) recognized the challenge of "developing culturally sensitive service options for all caregiver populations" (p. 6). In line with that, the Administration on Aging (2004) highlight a caregiving program in Tucson that is culturally and linguistically appropriate for its predominantly Mexican American population.

Funding for the family caregiver support programs at the state level is provided using a formula that takes into account the number of people over 70 in the state and is funded annually as a block grant. Authorization for the program ends in 2005. In fiscal year, 2005, the Administration on Aging provided approximately $155 million to states for NFCSP programs (Administration on Aging, 2005). While this program lends itself well to the development and delivery of innovative caregiver support program, Feinberg and Newman (2004) argue that the funding level is meager. When contrasted with the amount of federal money spent on nursing care, it is indeed a meager sum. Further, the state matching requirements of federal funding for the NFCSP poses a major challenge for states in the face of their current budgetary constraints.

Medicaid Waiver Programs

Medicaid waiver programs provide another avenue by which federal policy may encourage family caregiving. Although historically a health insurance for low-income people, Medicaid funds a majority of the long term care services in the United States (39% in 1998), most of which takes place in nursing homes (Johnson & Sasso, 2000; Miller, 2005). Because social policy can influence the resource allocation and thus the

choices available, Montgomery and Feinberg (2003) argue that the un-
equal funding of institutional care limits the home and community-
based service (HCBS) choices available to people who need long-term
care. States may provide special "consumer directed" as well as home
and community-based services for persons who require these services
under two primary waiver programs: Section 1115 and Section 1915c of
the Social Security Act (U.S. House Committee on Ways and Means,
2004). Although these programs might help supplement the caregiving
efforts of family, eligibility for them are strictly based on the older adult
meeting the specific criteria for services. Indeed, these programs do not
take into account the caregivers' needs or abilities.

Section 1115. Section 1115 of the Social Security Act allows states to
implement Medicaid-funded programs that are not subjected to the
standard Medicaid requirements of comparability, statewide provision
of the program, or the ability to choose a provider (U.S. House Committee on Ways and Means, 2004).

One program that was developed under this waiver was the Cash and
Counseling Demonstration, a consumer-directed demonstration program. In 1999, the HCFA manual specifically allowed states to include
"consumer directed" services. "In such cases, the Medicaid beneficiary
may hire their own provider, train the provider according to their personal preferences, supervise and direct the provision of personal case
services, and if necessary, fire the provider." Family members are specifically excluded from this definition of personal care attendants if they
are legally responsible relatives (HCFA State Medicaid Manual, Section
4480). Depending upon the state in which this provision is implemented, payment may be made to relatives who are not financially responsible for the recipient's care (Stone & Keigher, 1994; HCFA State
Medicaid Manual, Section 4480). Tilly and Weiner (2001) found that
while a significant minority of older adults prefers consumer-directed
care, a significant majority of service providers question their abilities
to manage their own care. This might restrict the options and opportunities for frail older adults and their families.

An experimental study of Cash and Counseling services in Arkansas
between 1998-2001 found that participants who were able to choose their
caregiver were happier with the care they received, had fewer unmet
needs, and reported a higher quality of life (Foster, Brown, Philips,
Schore, & Carlson, 2003). It is important to note however that the data
relied heavily on reports from proxies. The average allowance that
participants received to pay for personal care assistance was $320 a
month, which paid for approximately 47 hours of services.

Further, a 2001 study of the Cash and Counseling Program in New Jersey of staff members of programs and state officials found that there were several obstacles to implementing a statewide cash and counseling program. Staff members had difficulty selling the program to older adults. The state also had difficulty recruiting agencies to provide consulting services to support and advise recipients on their plans. They also found that many participants named family members to act as representatives and these family members had been helping them prior to their joining the cash and counseling program. Lastly, participants did not find the restrictions on their cash spending unreasonable and that, with training and guidance, they were able to learn to hire, fire, supervise and train employees (Philips & Schneider, 2003).

Section 1915(c). The Home and Community Based Services (HCBS) waiver program, Section 1915(c) of Medicaid, was established in 1981, to encourage the provision of services to Medicaid recipients in non-institutional settings (Coleman, 1999). Participants have the choice to receive a waiver which enables them to receive care outside of an institutional setting or to receive institutional care. States have the authority to limit the number of people to whom they provide services through HCBS but people cannot be waitlisted for unduly long periods of time if they are found to be eligible for such services (Smith, 2004; Olmstead v. L.C., 1999). Designed to "reduce the institutional bias in the Medicaid program. . .," this waiver program provides for the coverage of medical and non-medical services to people who require long-term care (U.S. House Committee on Ways and Means, 2004, p. 15-Medicaid-44). Beginning in 1999, every state had at least one HCBS waiver program and such programs were responsible for approximately 16.5% of all long term care services Medicaid provided (Smith, O'Keefe, Carpenter et al., 2000; U.S. House Committee on Ways and Means, 2004). Waiver programs allow states to provide Medicaid services to people with higher incomes than what is traditionally allowed by Medicaid (42 CFR 440, 2000). Though this program has great potential, it is limited by the ability of an individual to fit within special programmatic criteria, available spaces in programs as well as the financial status of perspective recipients.

Minnesota's HCBS program provides services for several different populations using a single point of entry system, the county human service's agency. Regarding long-term care, the counties provide "intake, assessment, preadmission screening, and service authorization" (Smith, O'Keefe, Carpenter et al., 2000, p. 158). In this way, Minnesota can coordinate funding streams and direct recipients toward available appropriate services. This type of system provides families with clearer and better access to services but has been criticized for not addressing the specific needs of specialized populations (Smith, O'Keefe, Carpenter et al., 2000).

Texas has merged their 1915(c) waiver programs with 1915(b) waiver programs, which allow states to require that some Medicaid beneficiaries receive their benefits through managed care, and provides long term care for older adults under this program. All HMOs must assign participants with a case manager who must coordinate the care a participant will receive (Smith, O'Keefe, Carpenter et al., 2000). Combining Part 1915(b) with Part 1915(c) may lead to increased program flexibility which may result in the increased availability of services that are supportive to the family caregivers. However, traditionally, HMOs have resulted in the reduction of care as a cost saving measure and this may limit payments available to caregivers.

CAREGIVER ORGANIZATIONS INFLUENCING POLICY-MAKING: CHALLENGES, SUCCESSES AND THE FUTURE

In this section, we discuss the challenges facing the involvement of caregivers in caregiver organizations. We look at the successes that these organizations have achieved in their organizing efforts. We end this section with a discussion on the future on family caregiving policies in the U.S.

Challenges

There are many challenges to developing effective long term care policies in the United State, where both federal power and regulations that intervene with the private sphere may be looked upon skeptically. Further, like all other policy areas, current long-term care policies and provisions reflect the financing mechanisms that not only allow for service duplications but also service gaps.

One of the greatest challenges to creating supportive policies for caregiving comes from the nature of the American political system which requires the assent of many people and a couple branches of government (the Legislative and Executive branches) to pass new federal laws. To compound this challenge, the political philosophies of elected officials differ over the government's role and involvement in the formation of policies to protect vulnerable citizens. As a result of the nature of the U.S. political system, we often develop piecemeal solutions to address social problems.

Another challenge is that there is no cohesive interest group supporting caregiving policies. The challenge, as Wilson (1989) notes when describing majoritarian politics, politics regarding policies in which costs and benefits are distributed among many people, is that issues as diffuse as caregiving often lead to symbolic, weak policies. The Family and Medical Leave Act as well as the National Family Caregiver Support Program are cases in point. At present, the people whose interests might be served by improving national caregiving policy might include almost anyone, women, men, older adults, and adults with disabilities. Related to this challenge is that of recognition of the caregiving role. Walker, Pratt, and Eddy (1995) argue that caregiving tasks are not necessarily distinct from the mutual aid that is expected of family members. Indeed, evidence suggests that family caregivers are less likely to identify themselves as caregivers and are more likely to ground their identity in their familial role (O'Connor, 2002). For example, wife caregivers are more likely to see caregiving as an extension of their spousal responsibilities (Walker, Pratt, & Eddy, 1995). Thus, these women are less likely to be a part of an interest group which advocates for the development of policies to support their family caregiving role.

Another challenge to the possible role of the federal government in encouraging and supporting caregiving is the recent administration's challenge to federalism. Medicaid and National Family Caregiving are block grant programs. Though block grant programs provide states with greater flexibility to determine the services that they wish to provide, if the federal government chooses to reduce its role in public welfare, the amount of federal contribution and thus, the influence of these federal programs could be significantly decreased (Sparer, 1996). Despite the apparent need to increase federal funding of caregiving, we are faced with an increasing deficit and a trend toward de-federalizing benefits. In other words, it is unlikely that under our current political administration federal dollars will be increased to cover the costs of caregiving. Moreover, we are faced with the realities of cuts, between $14 and $20 billion, in Medicaid spending over the next five years (Parrott, Sherman, & Hardy, 2005). Of course, these cuts have serious consequences for the existing federal long-term care spending under Medicaid.

Yet another challenge facing caregiver organization is getting public support for policies that are sensitive to the caregivers' needs. Part of this challenge is in overcoming the public perception that caregiving is a private matter and that the government should not be involved in a fa-milial issue. The public does not always realize that caregiving can be potentially devastating to the caregivers' financial and psychological well-being. Tronto (1993) suggests that the current fragmentation of care policies serves to maintain the power of the privileged and that care activities are mainly completed by women and minorities. She further notes that "[C]are work is devalued," (p. 121) largely because it is con-sidered to be private work, primarily completed by women and public accomplishments, those traditionally done by men, are more valued. As a result of her analysis, it seems that the struggle to obtain government support for caregiving activities will be a largely uphill battle requir-ing a reframing of care as a more valued activity (Tronto, 1993). Silverstein and Parrott (2001) found that non-caregivers, though less supportive of governmental intervention, were more supportive of "noninvasive policy approaches" targeted at employment policies and tax relief for caregivers.

Strategies for Policy Advocacy

The passage of the FMLA in 1993 and NFCSP in 2000 represent the successes of various organizations across age and population groups working together to represent family caregivers. Coalition building is an important element in affecting change, and Haynes and Mickelson (2003) argue that a coalition of diverse groups might be potentially more powerful in bringing about policy changes. The National Alliance of Caregivers (NAC) represents an alliance of 40 national organizations that aim to support family caregivers and professionals serving them. The NAC has completed two national surveys on caregiving, which provide snapshot profiles of family caregivers, their care receivers, and also the impact of their caregiving. These reports are important in docu-menting the extent of family caregiver involvement in the U.S. long-term care system, as well as the cost that they bear in meeting the needs of the frail relatives.

In echoing the belief in coalition building, the NAC and Partnership for Caring (2001) proposed the creation of a caregiver empowerment group that strategically advocated on behalf caregivers' needs and de-veloping a legislative agenda. To this end, the Alzheimer's Association has successfully organized its membership, which includes family caregivers, with its annual public policy forum that offers participants the opportunity to hone their advocacy skills, create new and sustain networks with peers who are affected by or interested in Alzheimer's disease, and opportunities to visit and talk to their elected representatives. While the organization has been successful in generating public interest and support in Alzheimer's disease, specifically in securing funding for research on prevention and treatment of the disease, it is less successful in passing legislation that are supportive of caregivers of people with Alzheimer's disease.

Prior to successfully advocating for policies to support caregiving, advocates must develop a common identity among caregivers. Some strategies for helping caregivers develop this identity include group work and the use of the Internet.

Chadiha et al. (2004) identify storytelling as a useful strategy in raising awareness among caregivers of the similarities of their conditions. To this end, O'Connor (2002) found that a group experience for caregivers facilitated the members' construction and identification of themselves as caregivers. This is an important challenge to overcome because the beginning of a social movement in affecting policy changes begins with the development of consciousness of the problem or need (Haynes & Mickelson, 2003). Additionally, O'Connor (2002) reports that by using groups, members begin to realize that some of their problems stem from situational circumstances rather than personal circumstances.

The Internet may also provide opportunities for caregivers to develop a group identity. The Internet may allow them to participate in discussion forums and to be policy activists without worrying about arranging for alternative caregiving arrangements. However, there is a portion of senior citizens who do not use the Internet and thus, do not have access to these services. The AARP has a useful on-line service that provides information discussing caregiving options. These options include information on caregiver support, long-term care financing, help with home care, housing options, and caregiving for adult children. Caregivers can participate in an on-line discussion by posting their comments, questions, and responses on a web-based discussion board. Similarly, the Family Caregiver Alliance maintains a website that provides caregiver fact sheets, and research reports. Additionally, the Alliance has an on-line caregiver discussion group in the format of a list serve for caregivers to talk, share ideas, problem solve, strategize, and provide support for each other. These on-line forums can and do serve many functions including identity building among family caregivers, and they may become useful tools for advocacy work.

The Future

With the projected growth in the proportion and absolute numbers of the older population in the U.S., policies pertaining to the well-being of older people, including long-term care policies, will become increasingly important. Lynch and Estes (2001) argue that the demand for long-term care can affect many spheres. They argue that employers will have to deal with worker productivity and health and social services will have to deal with increase demands for these services related to long-term care. As we mentioned earlier, caregivers and their families will be affected at varying degrees by whatever policy measures that are undertaken. From their analyses of various national datasets, Arno, Levine, and Memmott (1999) estimated that we could expect to pay between $115 billion to $288 billion in 1997 if we were to purchase the care provided by families in the marketplace. The NAC and Partnership for Caring (2001) state that the experience of "caregiving should not be personally and financially devastating" to caregivers and their families (p. 1). Employed caregivers are likely to experience a loss in their wage wealth–defined as the present value of lifetime wages calculated as of the date of retirement–as well as a loss in their retirement income (National Alliance for Caregiving and the National Center on Women and Aging at Brandeis University, 1999). This loss in wages and future benefits can have long-term effects on the financial well being of some caregivers when they face their own retirement. While some observers balk at the monetization of caregiving, Vladeck (2004) argues that policy discourse in the U.S. inevitably centers on the issue that is related to funding. Change agents and ultimately, policymakers need to realize that caregiver-supportive policies are investments in the population (Foster & Brizius, 1993). As such, policies on caregiving must consider the economics of caregiving (Harrington, 2000).

By not including caregiving in the general political discourse, the needs of caregivers are often ignored by federal policy. For example, caregivers are affected by social security policy. By focusing the current discussion of social security reform on the future insolvency of the social security trust funds, we are ignoring the real threats that many employed caregivers currently face should they reduce their work hours or leave their job because of their caregiving demands. For these caregivers, more time spent caring for frail relatives may mean less time spent in their paid employment which may jeopardize their own Social Security benefits, both in the amount and their eligibility. Many have recommended the need to ensure that caregivers are not penalized for leaving paid employment in response to higher caregiving demands, in proposing that the government give Social Security credits to account for lost years of caregivers' employment due to caregiving demands (Arno, Levine, & Memmott, 1999; Feinberg & Newman, 2004; Older Women's League, 1999).

Long-term care policies, which support family caregiving efforts by allowing payments to family caregivers, such as the Cash and Counseling Programs in Arkansas, have been successful in increasing consumer satisfaction. Service providers need to work to overcome their biases in making consumer direct programs available for older adults, who can benefit from the autonomy and independence in hiring, firing, and training their caregivers. Further, other Medicaid Waiver programs have enabled older adults who qualify for nursing home care to receive these services in their communities, which can complement the efforts of family caregivers. As such, these programs need to be expanded for frail older adults.

Although a number of organizations have been organizing to bring about family-friendly long-term care policies, Lynch and Estes (2001) assert that the chances of any major reform in these policies are slim in the light of the current political and economic climate. Despite this bleak outlook, coalition building needs to continue among caregiver organizations in building a common advocacy platform for family caregivers. Montgomery and Feinberg (2003) argue that the recognition and support of the informal network in their caregiving efforts should be an underlying principle in policy making. Indeed, formal home care services not only enable frail older adults to meet the challenges of daily living, they should also support and complement the efforts of family caregivers (Caro, 2001).

CONCLUSION

While family caregivers bear much of the responsibilities of providing essential in-kind services to their frail older relatives, long-term care policies have either been more symbolic in recognizing the contributions of family caregivers or have focused entirely on paid services. In this paper, we discussed the arbitrary bifurcation of the private and public spheres, where caregiving is often viewed as a private family matter that's beyond the purview of governmental intervention. We believe that this perception needs to change in the light of the permeability between the so-called spheres. While policies such as the FMLA, NFCSP, and Medicaid Waiver Programs make provisions for the direct and indirect support of family caregivers, the funding cuts and strict eligibility criteria have limited the availability, accessibility and acceptability of these programs to many family caregivers.

Caregiver organizations have made a number of significant advances in the policy-making arena, especially when we consider the challenges inherent in the policy-making process. To be sure, there are many challenges ahead that will make the creation of comprehensive long-term care policies that are sensitive to the needs of both the care receivers and family caregivers a difficult process. Notwithstanding these challenges, we reiterate the need to highlight the contributions of family caregivers and the potential costs that they bear in the discussion of long-term care policy making. Policy discussions that do not consider the economic contributions and cost of caregiving can potentially have little or no effect in supporting the efforts of caregivers. In addition, we reiterate the need for family caregivers to develop a coherent identity and an effective voice in the lobbying process. Without such a voice, their needs are likely to be left symbolically rather than effectively addressed.

REFERENCES

Administration of Aging. *Administration on Aging: FY 2006 President's Budget*. Department of Health and Human Services. Retrieved on March 10, 2005 at http://www.aoa.dhhs.gov/about/legbudg/current_budg/budget-request_table.pdf

Administration of Aging, United States Department of Health and Human Services. (2004). *The Older Americans Act National Family Caregiver Support Program (Title III-G $ Title VI-G): Compassion in Action* [Electronic Version]. Available on-line: http://www.aoa.gov/prof/aoaprog/caregiver/careprof/progguidance/resources/FINAL%20NFCSP%20Report%20July22,%202004.pdf

Albert, S. M. (2004). Beyond ADL-IADL: Recognizing the full scope of family caregiving. In C. Levine (Ed.), *Family caregivers on the job: Moving beyond ADLs and IADLs* (pp. 99-122). New York: United Hospital Fund of New York.

Arno, P. S., Levine, C., & Memmott, M. M. (1999). The economic value of informal caregiving. *Health Affairs, 18*(2), 182-188.

Bengtson, V. L., Giarusson, R., Silverstein, M., & Wang, H. (2000). Families and intergenerational relationships in aging societies. *Hallym International Journal of Aging, 2* (1), 3-10.

Caro, F. G. (2001). Asking the right questions: The key to discovering what works in home care. *The Gerontologist, 41*(3), 307-308.

Centers for Medicare and Medicaid Services. (2005). *National Health Expenditures, 2003* [Electronic Version]. Available on-line: http://www.cms.hhs.gov/statistics/nhe/default.asp

Chadiha, L. A., Adams, P., Biegel, D. E., Auslander, W., & Gutierrez, L. (2004). Empowering African American women informal caregivers: A literature synthesis and practice strategies. *Social Work, 49* (1), 97-108.

Coleman, N. (1999). *Trends in Medicaid Long Term Care Spending.* [Electronic Version] American Association of Retired Citizens. Retrieved on March 21, 2005 from http://research.aarp.org/health/dd38_trends.html#community.

Commission on the Family and Medical Leave and U.S. Women's Bureau. (1996). *A workable balance: Report to Congress on family and medical leave policies.* Washington, DC: Author.

Family and Medical Leave Act. (1993). PL 103-3, 29 CFR §825 (1995).

Feinberg, L. F. & Newman, S. L. (2004). A study of 10 states since the passage of the National Family Caregiver Support Program: Policies, Perceptions, and Program Development. *The Gerontologist, 44*(6), 760-769.

Feinberg, L. F. & Newman, S. (2004). *Family caregiving and long-term care: A crucial issue for America's families.* San Francisco: Family Caregiver Alliance.

Feinberg, L. F., Horvath, J., Hunt, G., Plooster, L., Kagan, J., Levine C. et al. (2003). *Family caregiving and public policy: Principles for change.* Available on-line: www.caregiver,org.

Foster, S. E. & Brizius, J. A. (1993). Caring too much? American women and the nation's caregiving crisis. In J. Allen & A. Pifer (Eds.), *Women on the front lines: Meeting the challenge of an aging America* (pp. 47-73). Washington, DC: Urban Institute.

Foster, L., Randall, B., Phillips, B., Schore, J., & Carlson, B. (2003). Improving the quality of Medicaid personal assistance through consumer direction. *Health Affairs, 22*(1), 162-176.

FoxGrage, W., Coleman, B., & Blancato, R. B. (2001). *Federal and State policy in family caregiving: Recent victories but uncertain futures.* San Francisco: Family Caregiving Alliance.

Glass, J. L. & Estes, S. B. (1997). The family responsive workplace. *Annual Review of Sociology, 23,* 289-313.

Harrington, M. (1999). *Care and equality: Inventing a new family politics.* New York: Routledge.

Haynes, K. S. & Mickelson, J. S. (2003). *Affecting change: Social workers in the political arena* (5th ed.). Boston: Allyn and Bacon.

Herd, P. & Meyer, M. H. (2002). Care work: Invisible civic engagement. *Gender and Society, 16*(5), 665-688.

Johnson, R. W. & Sasso, A. T. L. (2000). *Parental care at midlife: Balancing work and family responsibilities near retirement.* Brief Series 9. Washington, DC: Urban Institute.

Lechner, V. M. & Neal, M. B. (1999). The mix of public and private programs in the United States: Implications for employed caregivers. In. V. M. Lechner & M. B. Neal (Eds.), *Work and caring for the elderly: International perspectives* (pp. 120-139). Philadelphia: Brunner/Mazel.

Levine, C. & Hart, A. (2004). Doing whatever needs to be done: Caregivers' perspective on ADLs and IADLs. In C. Levine (Ed.), *Family caregivers on the job: Moving beyond ADLs and IADLs* (pp. 1-36). New York: United Hospital Fund of New York.

Linsk, N. L., Keigher, S. M., Simon-Rusinowitz, L., & England, S. E. (1992). *Wages for caring: Compensating family care of the elderly*. New York: Praeger.

Lynch, M. & Estes, C. L. (2001). The underdevelopment of community-based services in the U.S. long-term care system. In C. L. Estes & Associates (Eds.), *Social policy and Aging: A critical perspective* (pp. 201-215). Thousand Oaks, CA: Sage Publications.

McGovern, P. & Matter, D. (1992). Work and family: Competing demands affecting worker well-being. *AAIHN Journal, 40*(1), 24-35.

Medicaid Home and Community Based Services. (2000). Health Care Financing Administration. 42 CFR §440-441.

Miller, E. A. (2002). State discretion and Medicaid program variation in long-term care: When is enough, enough? In G. G. Caro & R. Morris (Eds.), *Devolution and Aging Policy* (pp. 15-35). New York: The Haworth Press.

Montgomery, A. & Feinberg, L. F. (2003). *The road to recognition: International review of public policies to support family and informal caregiving*. San Francisco: National Center on Caregiving, Family Caregiver Alliance.

National Alliance for Caregiving & AARP. (1997). *Family caregiving in the U.S.: Findings from a national survey (Final Report)*. Washington, DC: Author.

National Alliance for Caregiving & AARP. (2004). *Caregiving in the U.S.* [Electronic version]. Available on-line at: www.caregiving.org/04finalreport.pdf

National Alliance for Caregiving and the National Center on Women and Aging at Brandeis University. (1999). *The MetLife Juggling Act Study*. New York: Metropolitan Life Insurance Company.

National Association of State Units on Aging. (2003). *The aging network implements the National Family Caregiver Support Program* [Electronic Version]. Available on-line: www.nasua.org.

O'Connor, D. L. (2002). Toward empowerment: Revisioning family support groups. *Social Work with Groups, 25*(4), 37-56.

Older Americans Act: National Family Caregiver Support Program (2000). PL 106-501.

Older Women's League. (2001). *Mother's Day Report*. Washington, DC: Author.

Olmstead v. L. C., 527 U.S. 581 (1999).

Organization for Economic Co-operation and Development (OECD). (1996). *Caring for frail elderly people: Policies in evolution* (Social Policy Studies, No. 19). Paris: Author.

Parrott, S., Sherman, A., & Hardy, B. (2005). *House budget resolution would require much deeper cuts in key low income programs than Senate budget plan* [Electronic Version]. Washington, DC: Center on Budget Policy and Priorities. Available on-line: http://www.cbpp.org/pubs/health.htm.

Philips, B. & Schneider, B. (2003). *Enabling Personal Preference: The Implementation of the Cash and Counseling Demonstration in New Jersey* [Electronic Version]. Washington, D. C: Office of Disability, Aging and Long-term Care, United States Department of Health and Human Services. Available on-line: http://aspe.hhs.gov/daltcp/reports/enablepp.pdf

Silverstein, M. & Parrott, T. M. (2001). Attitudes towards government policies that assist informal caregivers: The link between personal troubles and public issues. *Research on Aging, 23*(3), 349-374.

Smith, G. (2004). *Status Report: Litigation Concerning Home and Community Based Services for People with Disabilities* [available on-line]. Portland, OR: Human Services Research Institute. Available at: http: http://www.hsri.org/index.asp?id=news.

Smith, G., O'Keeffe, J., Carpenter, L., Doty, P., Kennedy, G., Burwell, B., Mollica, R., & Williams, L. (2000). *Understanding Medicaid Home and Community Services: A Primer.* George Washington University and the U.S. Department of Health and Human Services. Retrieved on March 30, 2005 at http://aspe.hhs.gov/daltcp/reports/primer.htm.

Sparer, M. (1996). *Medicaid and the limits of state health reform.* Philadelphia: Temple University Press.

Stone, R. I. & Keigher, S. M. (1994). Toward an equitable universal caregiver policy: The potential of financial support for family caregivers. *Journal of Aging and Social Policy, 6*(1/2), 57-75.

Stone, R. I., Cafferata, G. L., & Sangl, J. (1987). Caregivers of the frail elderly: A national profile. *The Gerontologist, 27,* 616-626.

Tilly, J. & Weiner, J. M. (2001). *Consumer-directed home and community services: Policy issues.* Washington, DC: The Urban Institute.

Tronto, J. (1993). *Moral Boundaries: A Political Argument for an Ethic of Care.* NY: Routledge.

United States House of Representatives, Committee on Ways and Means. (2004). *The Green Book.* [Electronic Version] Available on-line: http://waysandmeans.house.gov/Documents.asp?section=813

Vladeck, B. C. (2004). You can't get there from here: Dimensions of caregiving and dementias of policymaking. In C. Levine (Ed.), *Family caregivers on the job: Moving beyond ADLs and IADLs* (pp. 123-137). New York: United Hospital Fund of New York.

Walker, A. (1983). Care for elderly people: A conflict between women and State. In J. Finch & D. Groves (Eds.), *A labour of love: Women, work and caring* (pp. 106-128). London: Routledge and Kegan Paul.

White-Means, S. I. & Thornton, M. C. (1990). Ethnic differences in the production of informal home health care. *The Gerontologist, 30,* 758-768.

Wilson, J. Q. (1995). *Political Organizations.* Princeton, NJ: Princeton University Press.

Wisensale, S. (2003). Two Steps Forward, One Step Back: The Family and Medical Leave Act as Retrenchment Policy. *Review of Policy Research, 20*(1) 135-151.

Examining Fiscal Federalism, Regionalization and Community-Based Initiatives in Canada's Health Care Delivery System

Pierre-Gerlier Forest
Howard A. Palley

INTRODUCTION

This study focuses on the ability of Canadian provinces to shape in different ways the development of various provincial health care delivery systems within the constraint of the mandates of the federal Canada Health Act of 1984 and the fiscal revenues that the provinces receive if they comply with these mandates. In so doing it will examine the operation of Canadian federalism with respect to the health care delivery system.

This study posits a comparative analysis framework in order to facilitate an understanding of the dimensionality of provincial health care delivery systems. Three sets of relationships will be "dealt with" in various ways in the illustrated area of provincial health care system development which is examined: that is, the case of provincial regionalization of the delivery of health care services in various provinces. Regionalization is often characterized by community-focused health care programs and policies. The three sets of relationships touched upon are: First, the levels of government and the nature of their involvement in public policy concerning the provincial health care delivery systems. The second area dealt with is understanding of the factors influencing provincial governments' political dispositions to act in various directions and the third is to take into account the factors influencing the "timing" of particular decisions (Heisler & Peters, 1977; also see Brown, 1998; Marse & Paulus,

2003; Wessen, 1999). A fourth area noted by Heisler and Peters (1977) is the nature and characteristics of public and private sector activities in health care and other areas of social policy. While the evolving nature of public and private sector health care delivery activities within Canada's provincial and territorial systems is a significant public policy matter in the Canadian context, due to the space limitations of this article, they are not addressed herein.

FEDERALISM AND THE CANADA HEALTH ACT

The functioning of Canadian federalism in the area of health care service delivery is characterized by a competition between national fiscal power and the formal constitutional responsibility of the provinces to provide for provincial health care. This relationship is a stipulation of the initial Canadian constitution, the British North American Act of 1867, and the more recent Constitution of 1982 (Heuglin, 1986).

Under the Canada Health Act of 1984, in order for the provinces to receive full federal financial contributions (fiscal federalism), provincial programs must provide for the delivery of required health services. They must also meet criteria of public (non-profit) administration, comprehensiveness, universality, portability and accessibility. In addition, provincial "extra-billing" and user charges for health services are not permitted. Basic insured services which must be provided by the provinces as a condition of financial participation, as defined by the Canada Health Act, consist of all necessary hospital services, physician services and surgical dental services performed in a hospital. In addition under the Act, such provincial health insurance plans may provide for a number of "extended health services" including pharmaceuticals, nursing home care and in-home care in the provincial health care budgets (Maslove, 1998; Palley & Forest, 2004; Palley, 2000; Palley, 1987).

The federal/provincial relationship in health care service delivery has been viewed as "cooperative federalism," "collaborative federalism" or "partnership." "Cooperative federalism" implies cooperation between federal, provincial and territorial levels of government but with the initiative and financial leverage exerted by federal officials (Cameron & Simeon, 2002). "Collaborative federalism" or "partnership" assumes a more co-equal, provincial-territorial and federal relationship–a relationship closer to "codetermination" (Cameron & Simeon, 2002; Courchene, 1994; Rasmussen, 2001; White, 2002). While the federal/territorial relationship is constitutionally one of federal primacy, in functional terms the federal government usually operates in a "cooperative" or "collaborative" relationship with the territories with respect to the delivery of health care services. Thus, regardless of the particular nuance applicable in a particular situation, the federal/provincial-territorial relationship involves the facilitation of the delivery of health services in the provinces by joint meetings and other exchanges resulting in cooperative relationships and health policy developments (including federal funding decisions) between federal and provincial governmental officials (Adams, 2001; Heuglin, 2003; O'Reilly, 2001). Nevertheless recently, federal and provincial authorities often have been in adversarial postures (Adams, 2001; Boase, 2001; Fierlback, 2001; Grey, 1998). To some extent the federal policy of providing asymmetrical "equalization payments" to enable poorer provinces to achieve equitable regional health care services has contributed to these strains (Bird, 1994; O'Reilly, 2001). The "have" provinces feel they could make use of more revenue to meet citizen demands on the health care delivery system while the "have not" provinces feel that the federal government should be more generous in providing them with revenues. Quebec also is, in some situations, in an asymmetric relation with the anglophone provinces and the federal government and in some situations in a symmetric relationship. For instance in the September 2000 meeting of provincial premiers and federal officials, Quebec agreed with the Social Union Framework Agreement health accord but not the accord on early childhood development (Cameron & Simeon, 2002; for a discussion of the complexities of regional and cultural asymmetries in a federal state, see Swenden, 2002).

Meeting provincial obligations regarding the delivery of health services has been complicated by the fact that in the decade after the passage of the Canada Health Act, the average level of federal spending for health care in the provinces declined from "in the neighborhood" of 33 percent to 24 percent (Commission on the Future of Health Care in Canada, 2002). Faced with criticism from provincial governments in 1999, the level of federal funding was increased. The federal government has added an additional $11.5 billion (Canadian) of health care funding to the provinces for fiscal years 2000 through 2005 (Simpson, 1999). It has since added additional funds so that $34.8 billion (Canadian) will be added for 2003 through 2008 (Finance Canada, 2003a,b). Federal sources anticipate that this should return the average federal level of spending for health care in the provinces to the 37 percent level–if one includes tax points given by the federal government to the provinces in 1977 under the Established Programs Financing Act (Finance Canada,

2004; also see Finance Canada, 2005). (If one includes direct federal support for health care, the total federal contribution to national public health spending is about 40 percent [also see Finance Canada, 2004].) Furthermore, a September, 2004 First Ministers' Meeting will add an additional $41.2 billion (Canadian) over a 10 year period (Spurgeon, 2004). It is, in part, within this context that a movement for provincial health care reform has taken place.

THE SIGNIFICANCE OF FISCAL FEDERALISM

While the Canadian Health Act establishes federal conditions intended to secure a measure of equality regarding the right to health care for all Canadians regardless of province or territory of residence, the possibility of withdrawal of federal funds is a mechanism used to secure compliance with national requirements. Often simply a federal announcement of concern with a prospective provincial action deemed in violation of such national requirements is enough to secure compliance with the Canada Health Act. The different pressures and tensions of fiscal federalism are reflected, to some extent, in the political history of the changing nature of fiscal arrangements affecting the delivery of health care services. A brief review of such arrangements reveals continuing adjustments in the structure of fiscal federalism.

In 1977, the federal government replaced earlier targeted cost-sharing arrangements with a block grant of federal funds that was transferred to the provinces to assist in funding health care and post-secondary education under an Established Programs Financing (EPF) arrangement. This EPF arrangement distributed funds on an equal per capita basis to the provinces and it included both cash transfers and "tax point" equalization (tax transfers to the provinces). Provinces received fixed federal funding and essentially were to absorb other increases in health care (and post-secondary education) expenditures while at the same time being bound to federal conditions which were explicated in the Canada Health Act, as well as earlier federal statutes. Violations of these federal stipulations would result in financial penalties (Palley & Forest, 2004).

Initially, the EPF formula was calculated on the basis of GNP per capita growth; with federal fiscal deficits in 1986, it was reduced to GNP per capita growth minus two percent. In 1990, the federal EPF formula was frozen. With respect to fiscal federalism, there was a perception that EPF did not workout due to two reasons: the lack of federal "visibility" and activity commensurate with federal fiscal effort and the lack of federal financial contribution to the provinces vis-à-vis federal mandates under the Canada Health Act (Banting, Brown, & Courchene, 1994). This situation created a good deal of tension in negotiations between Ottawa and the provinces and undermined what had been considered a regime of intergovernmental "cooperative federalism" (Banting, Brown, & Courchene, 1994, p. 3). In 1995, the federal government proposed a replacement for the EPF arrangement along with the existing federal/provincial cost-sharing arrangement for means-tested social assistance (the Canadian Assistance Plan) into a super block grant, the Canada Health and Social Transfer grant (CHST) (Maioni & Maino, 2000). This mechanism represented an attempt to give provinces more flexibility in developing their budgets. The CHST initially substantially reduced the cash portion of the federal transfers available to the provinces which led critics to view this arrangement as a fiscal "shortfall" which threatened the federal government's ability to enforce the existing national requirements of the Canada Health Act (Maslove, 1998). Several provinces began to challenge Ottawa's role in the mandating of health care services.

In response to such criticisms, a five year federal cash floor was introduced in 1998 starting at $12.5 billion (Canadian) rising to $14.5 billion (Canadian) in 1999-2000–including a supplement of $2 billion (Canadian) targeted for health programs. In 1999, a new federal Equalization Payment was established to eliminate existing inter-provincial disparities with respect to health care programs (O'Reilly, 2001).[1] In 1999, under the CHST, all provinces, except Ontario, Alberta, and British Columbia could utilize funds under the Equalization Program to pay for health care services. Finally, in September 2000, the provinces negotiated a $23.4 billion (Canadian) health funding arrangement–with few conditions attached (O'Reilly, 2001). In February 2003, another agreement promised an additional $13.5 billion (Canadian) federal contribution to health care funding. In November 2003, the federal government offered the provinces an additional $2 billion (Canadian) in new health care funding fulfilling an agreement reached at the February, 2003 (Federal/Provincial) First Ministers' Health Accord (Finance Canada, 2003a; Cordon, 2003). Some of these revenues went into a special fund for diagnostic equipment, medical technology and investment to generally help the provinces upgrade their medical equipment. In the face of continuing complaints by the provincial governments that federal contribution to provincial health care services were insufficient to deal with current needs, as we have noted earlier, a new agreement was reached following a First Ministers' Meeting in September, 2004 that will cost the federal government an additional $41.2 billion (Canadian) (Spurgeon, 2004).

Among the goals of the agreement reached are reduction of patients' waiting times for access to health care services. The provincial premiers and territorial leaders in return agreed to set up national targets for medically acceptable waiting times in the area of treatment of cancer, heart disease, and for diagnostic imaging, joint replacement and sight restoration (Spurgeon, 2004). The provinces would establish separate benchmarks by individual province. They would also set targets for bringing down waiting times in their own jurisdictions. This information would be transmitted to the federal level which would utilize such information in establishing national suggested "targets" with respect to waiting times (Laghi et al., 2004). In addition, the agreement calls for increased federal funding to achieve an increase in the number of health professionals and particularly primary care physicians and for increasing funding for northern aboriginal communities (Spurgeon, 2004). It also calls for increased availability of short-term home care and hospice services; the development of a pharmaceutical plan to cover patients for illnesses with very high treatment costs, plus a new immunization program for children. At this meeting, Quebec secured a separate agreement which allows that province to develop its own plan for reducing waiting times and to develop its own drug formulary. However it would share with the other provinces and, indirectly, with the federal government such matters as its benchmarks for measuring improvement in waiting times, its measures taken to improve the provision of home care, access to drugs and for the prevention of chronic illness (Spurgeon, 2004).

One problem with the equalization transfer arrangements previously noted, was that, until the separation of Health Transfers from Social Transfers in April, 2004, there was no certainty as to what proportion of total CHST federal transfers had actually been apportioned by the provinces and territories to health programs as there was no specific targeting requirement in this program (Adams, 2001). In fiscal year 2004-2005, only Ontario and Alberta were not eligible to receive equalization funds (Finance Canada, 2005).

Such equalization funds flowed directly into provincial general revenues.[2] Of total federal revenue transfers for fiscal year 2004-2005, 80 percent was allocated through the CHST while 20 percent was derived from equalization payments. In Newfoundland and Labrador, 48 percent of federal transfers for health care and social services were distributed through the CHST and 52 percent was derived from equalization funds. In Quebec, 71 percent of federal funds for health and social services was received from the CHST and 29 percent was received from equalization payments (Finance Canada, 2004, 2005). Such "extra" benefits for poorer provinces are considered to be "asymmetrical" federal payments which are, in effect, regional transfers from richer to poorer areas which are viewed as maintaining "the 'glue' of nationhood" (Bird, 1994, p. 301). (The figures for fiscal year 2004-2005 involve a CHST/CHT/CST estimation process; other federal contributions specifically to health care are the Health Reform Transfer, Waiting Times Reduction and Territorial Formula Financing.) Nevertheless, increasingly demands for more health care services within the provinces has led both to continuing requests for additional federal funding and pressure for organizational reforms within the provincial health care systems. Also, as aforementioned, in a move to create greater transparency with respect to identifying actual spending for health care delivery at the provincial level, as of April 1, 2004, the federal CHST has been supplemented by a separate Health Transfer and Social Transfer.

Some Current Issues Concerning Fiscal Federalism

Some current debates regarding the future of "fiscal federalism" are focused on:

1. The appropriate level of federal contribution to provincial health care funding. One issue which has arisen is whether a transfer of federal taxing authority from the federal government to the provinces and territories should be considered a federal revenue contribution to provincial and territorial health care services.
2. The appropriate balance regarding "tax points" and cash transfer payments from the federal government to the provinces and territories. A transfer system emphasizing "tax points" transferred to the provinces and territories weakens federal oversight of the health delivery system while one emphasizing federal cash transfers (with the possibility of withholding such transfers) strengthens federal oversight.
3. A third area of discussion is that of the reform and future structuring of the equalization formula to assist the poorer provinces. As a result of demands by the larger provinces, the federal government agreed to allocate block grant health care supplements on an equal per capita basis and, with respect to demands by the smaller and less prosperous provinces, to remove the equalization ceiling on

funding to allow greater funding of health care services in equalization receiving provinces. The smaller (and poorer) provinces also demanded changes in the equalization formula to reflect their greater reliance on equalization funds to support public services–including health care services.

These matters have been the topics of discussion and negotiation at recent meetings of Provincial and Territorial Ministers of Health (2000) and Provincial and Territorial Ministers of Finance (2001; Finance Canada, 2003a).

One illustrative case of the varied and distinctive development in the organization and delivery of health care services has been in the area of provincial (and territorial) regionalization of health care services (and related social services) within the federal system. The following is an account of developments with respect to regionalization of health care services.

HEALTH CARE REFORM
AND REGIONALIZATION OF SERVICES

The movement for health care reform throughout Canada in the late 1980s and 1990s has included demands for the regionalization of health care services within the provinces. However, in no case has this model encompassed the Swedish model of health care services in which a significant proportion of health and social services spending is based on local funding (Immergut, 1999). However, this future possibility has been suggested by some Canadian health policy analysts (Working Group Synthesis Report, 1997). In part, the movement for regionalization is the result of pressures from the federal level of government on the provinces and territories that they need to develop mechanisms to be less institution-based, more community-based and more efficient in terms of producing high quality health care services in a cost-effective manner.

Rather regionalization has been used as a device for shifting the priorities of health service funding from a vertical-base (particularly in the hospital sector) to a more horizontal, community-focused base encompassing preventive, habilitation and rehabilitation services, as well as long-term care and acute care services (Charles & Badgley, 1999; Deber, 1994; Fooks, 1999). Regionalization also has been viewed as a mechanism for improving management and accountability in provincial health systems (Deber & Swan, 1998; Fooks, 1999; Lomas, Woods, & Veenstra, 1997; Plain, 1997). However, in British Columbia, Saskatchewan and Nova Scotia, provincial regionalization had devolved management functions to an extent that there developed a danger of undermining of the notion of a provincial health delivery system (Hurley, Lomas, & Bhatia, 1994). The oft stated goal of such provincial regionalization is to increase the cost/effectiveness as well as the quality of health care delivery of services within the provinces and the territories.

Saskatchewan's regional health authorities have a somewhat unique history. As of October, 1995, two-thirds of its members were elected on the basis of universal suffrage from wards within each region; the remaining one-third of members are appointed. Direct election was eventually ended in the 2001-2002 period ("Provincial Overview Table," 2003). Significant numbers of the membership of Saskatchewan's regional authorities (49 percent) indicated in a 1997 survey that regional devolution represented the provincial government's desire to "offload" tough budgetary decisions (Dickenson, Kouri, Williams, Hurley et al., 2001).

Such health regions were "realigned" in 2003 in a reorganization in Saskatchewan that reduced 32 health districts to 12. This reorganization has raised some concerns regarding continued representation from small rural communities (Driver, 2003). A similar survey concerning regional devolution in Alberta found that 67 percent of its regional health authority members also held the view that such devolution was motivated by the provincial government's concern with "offloading" difficult budgetary decisions (Dickenson, Kouri, Williams, Hurley et al., 2001).

This restructuring was accelerated by the federal cutbacks in support of health care services in the late 1980s and the 1990s as well as the general need of provincial governments to address serious fiscal deficits (Grey, 1998). (Yet in spite of such reforms, hospital care remains the largest health care expenditure area in Canada. In 2004, hospital care expenditures amounted to $38,9 billion Canadian–29.9 percent of total health care expenditures; this was followed by drug expenditures of $21.8 billion Canadian–or 16.7 percent of total health care expenditures [Canadian Institute for Health Information (CIHI), 2004]. Nevertheless the reduction of hospital costs as a percentage of health care expenditures and the increase in drug costs as a percentage of health care expeditures indcates that increasingly health care services take place on an in-home and community-based basis.) In all provinces except Ontario the creation of regional and community health boards for purposes of resource allocation and direct management of facilities have been a characteristic of health care reorganization in the 1990s (Redden, 1999). Regionalization in Ontario through District Health Councils has been limited to recommendary authority concerning the organization of health services and provision for consultation with local populations. This "restructuring" has often preceded decisions regarding the distribution of health resources made within communities and the distributional equity of such decisions.

The 1997 Lomas analysis provides a number of interesting observations regarding regionalization. Commenting on Alberta's attempt to use such regional authorities as a way of rationalizing budget cuts, he notes that Alberta's experience emphasizes the danger of a provincial government's over-relying on devolved authorities as buffers for local discontent. He further observes, that in this situation *in Alberta, the devolved, more locally-based regional authorities became critics of the provincial government, and added their authority to that of the citizenry's claims that the provincial health system is underfunded* (Lomas, 1997).

Regarding provinces with two-tiered structures of regional and community health authorities, such as exist in British Columbia, Manitoba and Nova Scotia, some confusion over relative roles and responsibilities occurred. Nevertheless, since budgetary authority in these systems lies with the regional level, hospital integration and rationalization remained the primary thrust, rather than the concern with coordinating and providing home care, community services and the location of physician offices (Lomas, 1997). In provinces with only regional boards, such as Alberta, Quebec and New Brunswick, a significant problem has been the apparent lack of resources in some areas needed to provide an equitable level of primary care, rehabilitative and other social support services in all regions (Boudreau, 1999).

Success in integrating social and human services beyond hospital rationalization requires that the regional boards have broad budgetary authority including the authority to regulate physicians' fees and drug pricing as well as to make budgetary determinations regarding social services as has been the case with Prince Edward Island's regional authorities (Lomas, 1997). *Such broader integration of community-based services is clearly a goal articulated by the statement of Manitoba's Regional Health Authorities.*
The statement expresses the sentiment that:

> *A regional model will more easily link prevention and promotion, alternative community-based care and actions on population health determinants into a seamless structure of service delivery than the current institution/physician-oriented system.* (our italics) (Regional Health Authorities of Manitoba, 2001, pp. 1-2)

Regionalization of provincial health services may be congruent with a high degree a centralized provincial control of health care services policy. The province of Quebec provides a good illustration of how centrally-determined health services policies have been budget-allocated, administered and managed at the regional and local level–but are constrained by budget determinations made centrally and by regional officials appointed centrally.

Quebec's Regional Health Boards have historically functioned alongside a system of parallel community public health departments and often have acted in concert with Quebec's local system of Centres Locaux des Services Communitaires (CLSCs). Quebec had established (initiated in 1968) a system of 160 nonprofit, community operated CLSCs (Béland, 1999a; Palley, 1987). The CLSCs offer at the primary care level, basic health and social services of both a preventive and curative nature and also rehabilitation and reintegration services to the population in the area served by the CLSC. However, Quebec's provincial government continues to oversee and evaluate CLSC programs and service delivery (Béland, 1999b; Palley & Forest, 2004; Soderstrom & Bozzini, 1994). With the closing and consolidation of hospitals in the 1990s, CLSCs were increasingly involved with community-based long-term care for the elderly (Cardwell, 1997; College des Médecines de Québec, 1998). Agreements in this area entered into by CLSCs have varied. Some have contracted out services to private nursing homes and home care agencies–both for-profit and non-profit agencies.

Also, CLSCs have had to retrain formerly hospital-based nurses for community care functions (Gottleib, 1999; Soderstrom, 1999; Soderstrom, Tousignant, & Kaufman, 1999). CLSCs are also increasingly involved in post-operative care in home care settings such as that of PRISMA (Program for Integrated Services for the Maintenance of Autonomy) in the Sherbrooke area and the Integrated Services Program in Quebec's Bois Francs area (Archambault & Bonin, 2001; Morin, 2002; PRISMA Program, 2002).

The role of the Regional Health Boards was further articulated under recent governmental reforms which had been recommended in 2001 by the *Report of the Commission for the Study of Health and Social Services* (The Clair Commission). This role was to budget-allocate, administer and implement policies within the constraints of budgetary decisions centrally determined at the provincial level (Chodos, 2001; Maioni, 2001). Following the recommendations of the Clair Commission's Report, the members of the Regional Health Boards were to be appointed by Quebec's provincial government from a list of names proposed by a local committee which in turn was composed of members appointed by the provincial government (Hawley-McDonald, 2002). Moreover the Regional Boards' administrators, as recommended by the Clair Commission Report, were to be appointed centrally, by Quebec's Minister of Health and Social Services, rather than elected by the Board's members.

Under this system, the development of integrated services (prevention, detection, cure and rehabilitation) for specified targeted groups (including the infirm elderly, mentally handicapped and chronically-ill) was budget-allocated by Regional Health Boards and coordinated by community-based CLSCs–although the Regional budgets were determined by Quebec's provincial government. This process involved CLSCs in serving as key institutions in the provision of social services–including a broad array of psycho-social services. Also, together with Regional Health Boards, the CLSCs assisted in monitoring the quality and performance of the long-term care system's facilities and services. However, as the administrators and members of these Boards were appointed centrally, it also gave more control to the Ministry of Health and Social Services in limiting the independence of these bodies (Kushner & Rachlis, 1998).

The Continuing Evolution of Regionalization in Quebec

Following the election of April, 2003 and the return of the Liberal Party to governance in Quebec, a health organization reform proposed in the political campaign was formalized in November, 2003 as *Bill 25, An Act Respecting Local Health and Social Service Network Development Agencies (agences de développements de réseaux locaux de services de santé et de services sociaux)*. This Bill was enacted into law in December, 2003. It provided that as of January 29, 2004, the Regional Boards were dissolved and on January 30, 2004 they were reconstituted as Local Health and Social Services Network Development Agencies. The previous boards of directors, presidents of the board and executive directors are reappointed in their continuing roles as members of the new development agencies.

The new charge of these agencies is to consult with localities and develop local "models of regroupment." That is, within two years, plans for local community-based networks of health and social services composed of CLSCs, hospitals and long-term care systems were to be organized in local geographical areas. These local networks would also be responsible for guaranteeing access of their populations to specialized and "superspecialized" (tertiary) services. Each area will provide integrated services under one board of directors. The former multiplicity of boards for various CLSCs, hospitals and long-term care systems would cease to exist. The plans for such "regroupment" would be developed within two years and would then be sent by the community-based Network Development Agencies to the Minister of Health and Social Services where they would need to be approved by the Ministry "with or without modifications." Upon acceptance of these plans, the Ministry would appoint provisional members of the local boards of directors who would serve for a two year period. The chief executive officer of these agencies also would be appointed by the Minister of Health and Social Services for no longer than a three year mandate. After the two year appointments to the various boards of directors, there would be local nominations for membership on the boards of directors which would lead to formal appointments by the Ministry to the local networks.

The hope is that these new local networks will be administratively and economically seamless organizations resulting in more functional, better coordinated and more economically efficient local health delivery systems. While this reform ended the former regionalization structure within two years, it retains the high degree of administrative accountability of "local community-based networks" to the Ministry of Health and Social Services and of centralized budgetary allocations. This reform created 95 local networks in the 18 regional districts. The restructuring is focused on improving the integration of services in local networks, mostly around primary care and specialized services. In this process, general hospital, long-term care centers and CLSCs have been merged into a new unit called a Centre de Santé et des Services Sociaux (CSSS). The CSSSs are also responsible for coordination of other care providers in their areas of jurisdiction in order to facilitate access to services and continuity of care for their respective populations (Fleury, 2006).

SOME CONCLUSIONS CONCERNING REGIONALIZATION

Regionalization may provide devolved but limited budgetary authority and management functions within the health care delivery system of various provinces. The arrangements of health care services under provincial systems of regionalization have been varied. Regionalization generally has been utilized as a device for attempting to shift some health care service funding from the institutional (hospital/nursing home) sector to a more horizontal, community-based and community-focused system emphasizing prevention and primary care, and habilitation and rehabilitation services. In a national and provincial health care delivery system with increasing budgetary problems, it has also often been viewed as a tool for "buffering" difficult allocation and management decisions by shifting them from the provincial level to the regional and community levels.

In some provinces, regionalization has devolved management to such an extent that regional equity and regional accountability regarding levels and quality of care have been undermined. In the case of Alberta, regional health authorities "unexpectedly" challenged provincial authorities to provide greater funding and resources for the provincial health care delivery system. In Quebec, centralized appointment and budgetary authority made it difficult for regional health authority board members to fight for regional equity in the provision of services under the health care delivery system. Also, current reforms of regionalization of the health care delivery system in Saskatchewan are aimed at creating wider geographic administrative units while reforms of regionalization in Quebec focus on creating smaller geographic administrative units. Thus, the results of "regionalization" have been as varied and unique as the political dynamics of the various provinces within the framework of overall national health care policies.

CONCLUSION

While fiscal federalism sets important constraints on provincial health care budgets, the Canadian constitutional prerogatives of the provinces have allowed the provinces to approach "regionalization" in a variety of ways–from an experiment in "democratization" and decentralization in Saskatchewan to a mechanism reinforcing centralized, administrative control with local, community-based implementation in Quebec. Also, a province can decide to "not regionalize" its overall health care delivery system as in the case of Ontario. Nevertheless, a general trend of regionalization across provinces has been the integration and consolidation of hospitals and a greater emphasis on the development of community-based and home-based health care and related social services with the goals of reducing hospital and other institutional costs and of providing a higher quality of health care services.

Thus, utilizing three dimensions of Heisler and Peters' framework as a general guide, we note that the Canadian health care delivery system remains a dynamic and varied one in terms of the levels of government involved in the delivery of health care services within a framework of fiscal federalism and in terms of the uniqueness of the provincial health care delivery systems within the federal system. This includes unique patterns of regionalization within provincial health care delivery systems that often emphasize increased community-based delivery of health care services. In addition, our examination of regionalization illustrates that political and governmental inputs at the federal level and within the various provinces are factors affecting the development of the policies and programs characterizing Canada's provincial (and territorial) health care delivery systems.

NOTES

1. Under the May, 1999 Social Union Framework Agreement between all provinces, except Quebec, as well as the Yukon and the Northwest Territories and the federal government, a three year agreement was reached whereby the federal government agreed not to introduce any new national programs unless a majority of the provinces agreed to accept them. The federal government also agreed that any new programs would only be initiated with federal funding. Furthermore, as an incentive to the provinces the federal government agreed to increase revenues to the provinces by several billion dollars, while Quebec has benefited from this funding, it did not formally join the social union agreement because the federal government dropped a provision which would have allowed provinces to back out of national programs but accept the federal financing that accompanied them if they were to substitute local programs which provided similar goals and standards (Adams, 2001; DePalma, 1999).

2. The following numbers have been rounded and adjusted to avoid double counting and therefore do not add up to 100 percent. Also, these numbers do not include the Health Reform Transfer.

REFERENCES

Adams, D. (2001). Canadian federalism and the development of national goals and objectives. In Adams, D. (Ed.), *Federalism, democracy and health policy in Canada* (pp. 61-105). Kingston, Ontario: School of Policy Studies, Institute of Intergovernmental Relations, Queen's University, McGill-Queen's University Press.

Archambault, C. & Bonin, L. (2001, October). *Réseau de services intègres aux Aines des Bois-Francs*, présentation de régie régionale, Sherbrooke, Québec.

Banting, K. G., Brown, D. M. & Courchene, T. J. (1994). The future of fiscal federalism: An overview. In Banting, K. G., Brown, D. M. & Courchene, T. J. (Eds.), *The future of fiscal federalism* (pp. 3-21). Kingston, Ontario: School of Policy Studies, Institute of Intergovernmental Relations, John Deutsch Institute for the Study of Economic Policy, Queen's University.

Béland, F. (1999a, May 14). Professor, Department of Health Administration, University of Montreal. *Interview*. Montreal, Quebec.

Béland, F. (1999b). Preventive and primary care access systems: CLSCs as neighbor-
    hood health and social service centers in Quebec. In Powell, F. D. & Wessen, A. F.
    (Eds.), *Health care systems in transition* (pp. 173-198). Thousand Oaks, CA: Sage
    Publications.
*Bill 25. An Act Respecting Local Health and Social Services Network Development
    Agencies* (2003). Quebec City, Quebec: Quebec Official Publisher.
Bird, R. M. (1994). A comparative perspective on federal financing. In Banting, K.G.,
    Brown, D. M. & Courchene, T. J. (Eds.), *The future of fiscal federalism* (pp. 35-52).
    Kingston, Ontario: School of Policy Studies, Institute of Intergovernmental Rela-
    tions, John Deutsch Institute for the Study of Economic Policy, Queen's University.
Boase, J. P. (2001). Federalism and the health facility fees challenge. In Adams, D.
    (Ed.), *Federalism, democracy and health policy in Canada* (pp. 17-59). Kingston,
    Ontario: School of Policy Studies, Institute of Intergovernmental Relations, Queen's
    University, McGill-Queen's University Press.
Boudreau, A. (1999, May 12). Directeur General. Régie Régionale de la Santé et Des
    Services Sociaux de l'Outaouais. *Interview*. Hull, Quebec.
Brown, L. D. (1998). "Exceptionalism as the rule? U.S. policy innovation and cross-
    cultural learning. *Journal of Health Politics, Policy and Law*, 23, 35-52.
Cameron, D. & Simeon, R. (2002). Intergovernmental relations in Canada: The emer-
    gence of collaborative federalism. *Publius: The Journal of Federalism*, 32, 49-67.
Canadian Institute for Health Information (CIHI). (2004). *National health expenditure
    trends 1975-2004*. Ottawa, Ontario, Canada.
Cardwell, M. (1997, March 26). Quebec City doctors not ready for massive changes.
    The Medical Post, pp. 1 & 33.
Charles, C. A. & Badgley, F. R. (1999). Canadian national health insurance: Evolution
    and unresolved policy issues. In Powell, F. D. & Wessen, A. F. (Eds.), *Health care
    systems in transition* (pp. 115-150). Thousand Oaks, CA: Sage Publications.
Chodos, H. (2001, February). *Quebec's health review (The Clair Commission)*. Ottawa,
    Canada: Political and Social Affairs Division, Research Branch of the Library of
    Parliament.
Collège des Medicines de Québec, Québec (QC). (1998, November). *Report by the
    task force of the reorganization of the health care system and the quality of medical
    services*. Quebec City, Quebec.
Commission on the Future of Health Care in Canada. (2002, November). *Building on
    values: The future of health care in Canada: final report*. Saskatoon, Saskatchewan.
Commission for the Study of Health and Social Services (The Clair Commission).
    (2001). *Report of the commission for the study of health and social services*. Quebec
    City, Quebec.
Cordon, S. (2003, November 3). Ottawa will drain federal surplus to offer provinces
    $2 billion more for health. *Canadian Press* from http:// www.regionalization.org,
    November 11, 2003.
Courchene, T. J. (1994). Canada's social policy deficit: Implications for fiscal federal-
    ism. In Banting, K. G., Brown, D. M. & Courchene, T. J. (Eds.), *The future of fiscal
    federalism* (pp. 83-122). Kingston, Ontario: School of Policy Studies, Institute of
    Intergovernmental Relations, John Deutsch Institute for the Study of Economic
    Policy, Queen's University.

Deber, R. B. (1994). Philosophical underpinnings of Canada's health care systems. In Lemco, J. (Ed.), *National health care: Lessons for the United States and Canada* (pp. 43-67). Ann Arbor: The University of Michigan Press.

Deber, R. B. & Swan, B. (1998). Puzzling issues in health care financing. In National Health Forum. *Striking a balance: Health care systems in Canada and elsewhere*, Vol. 4 (pp. 307-342). Sainte-Foy, Quebec: Editions MultiMondes.

DePalma, A. (1999, May 5). Ottawa and provinces (but not Quebec) in pact on national social programs. *The New York Times*, p. A6.

Dickinson, H., Kouri, D., Williams, J. I, Hurley J. et al. (2001). Devolution to democratic health authorities in Saskatchewan: An interim report. *Canadian Medical Association Journal*, 164, 343-347.

Driver, D. (2003, November 4). Health regions reorganized in Saskatchewan. *The Medical Post*, from http://www.regionalization.org, November 6, 2003.

Fierlbeck, K. (2001). Cost containment in health care: The federalism context. In Duane Adams, D. (Ed.), *Federalism, democracy and health policy in Canada* (pp. 131-178). Kingston, Ontario: School of Policy Studies, Institute of Intergovernmental Relations, Queen's University, McGill-Queen's University Press.

Finance Canada. (2003a, October). *Federal support for health care: The facts*. Ottawa, Ontario.

Finance Canada. (2003b). *Major federal transfers to provinces and territories*. Ottawa, Ontario.

Finance Canada. (2004, September). *Federal support for health care: The facts*. Ottawa, Ontario.

Finance Canada. (2005, March 31). *Major federal transfers to provinces and territories*. Ottawa, Ontario.

Fleury, M.-J. (2006, February 3). Adjunct Professor, Department of Psychiatry. Research Center of Douglas Hospital, McGill University. *E-Mail Communication*. Verdun, Quebec.

Fooks, C. (1999). Will power, cost control and health reform in Canada, 1987-1992. In Powell, F. D. & Wessen, A. F. (Eds.), *Health Care Systems in Transition* (pp. 151-172). Thousand Oaks, CA: Sage Publications.

Gottleib, L. (1999, May 14). Dean, School of Nursing, McGill University. *Interview*. Montreal, Quebec.

Grey, G. (1998). Access to medical care under strain: New pressures on Canada and Australia. *Journal of Health Politics, Policy and Law*, 23, 905-947.

Hawley-McDonald, G. (2002, September 24). Community Relations Agent, Régie Régionale de la Santé et des Services Sociaux de l'Outaouais. *Telephone Interview*. Hull, Quebec.

Heisler, M. O. & Peters, G. B. (1977). Towards a multidimensional framework for the analysis of social policy. *Annals of the American Academy of Political and Social Sciences*, 434, 60-69.

Heuglin, T. O. (1986). *Federalism and fragmentation: A comparative view of political accomodation*. Kingston, Ontario: Institute of Government, Queen's University.

Heuglin, T. O. (2003). Federalism at the crossroads: Old meanings, new significance. *Canadian Journal of Political Science*, 36, 275-294.

Hurley, J., Lomas, J. & Bhatia, V. (1994). When tinkering is not enough: Provincial reform to manage health care resources. *Canadian Public Administration*, 37, 490-514.

Immergut, E. (1999). Historical and institutional foundations of the Swedish health care system. In Powell, F. D. & Wessen, A. F. (Eds.), *Health care systems in transition* (pp. 201-204). Thousand Oaks, CA: Sage Publications.

Kushner, C. & Rachlis, M. (1998). Civic lessons: Strategies to increase consumer involvement in health care policy development. In National Health Forum, *Canada Health Action: Building a Legacy–Making Decisions: Evidence and Information*, Vol. 5 (pp. 295-338). Sainte-Foy, Quebec: Editions MultiMondes, 1998.

Laghi, B., Clark, C. & Fagan, D. (2004, September 16). The Medicare summit. *The Globe and Mail*, pp. 1 & 10.

Lomas, J. (1997). Devolving authority for health care in Canada's provinces: 4. Emerging issues and prospects. *Canadian Medical Association Journal*, 156, 817-823.

Lomas, J., Woods, J. & Veenstra, G. (1997). Devolving authority for health care in the Canadian provinces: 1. An introduction to the issues. *Canadian Medical Association Journal*, 156, 370-377.

Mahtre, S. L. & Deber, R. B. (1992). From equal access to health care to equitable access to health care: A review of Canadian provincial health commissions and reports. *International Journal of Health Services*, 22, 645-668.

Maioni, A. (2001, January 26). *"Emerging solutions": Quebec's Clair Commission Report and health care reform*. Montreal, Quebec: CPRN Backgrounder.

Maioni, A. & Maino, F. (2000, August 3). Fiscal federalism and health care reforms in Canada and Italy. Paper presented to the Annual Meeting of the International Political Science Association, Quebec City, Quebec.

Marse, H. & Paulus, A. (2003). Has solidarity survived? A comparative analysis of the effect of social health insurance reform in four European countries. *Journal of Health Politics, Policy and Law*, 28, 585-614.

Maslove, A. W. (1998). National goals and the federal role in health care. In National Health Forum, *Striking a Balance: Health Care System in Canada and Elsewhere* Vol. 4 (pp. 371-399). Sainte-Foy, Quebec: Editions MultiMondes.

Morin, P. (2002, March 21). Staff, PRISMA. *Telephone Interview*. Sherbrooke, Quebec.

O'Reilly, P. (2001). The Canadian health system landscape. In Adams, D. (Ed.), *Federalism, democracy and health policy in Canada* (pp. 107-129). Kingston, Ontario: School of Policy Studies, Institute of Intergovernmental Relations, Queen's University, McGill-Queen's University Press.

Palley, H. A. (1987). Canadian federalism and the Canadian health care program: A comparison of Ontario and Quebec. *International Journal of Health Services*, 17, 595-616.

Palley, H. A. (2000). An essay review comparing the U.S. and Canadian health care systems. *Journal of Health and Social Policy*, 11, 79-85.

Palley, H. A. & Forest, P.-G. (2004). Canadian fiscal federalism, regionalization, and the development of Quebec's health care delivery system. *New Global Development: Journal of International and Comparative Social Welfare*, 20, 87-96.

Plain, R. H. M. (1997). The role of health care reform in reinventing government. In Alberta. Bruce, C., Kneebone, R., & McKenzie, K. (Eds.), *A government reinvented:*

A study of Alberta's deficit elimination program (pp. 283-327). Toronto and New York: Oxford University Press.

PRISMA Program, website: www.pris,a-qc.ca, 2002.

Provincial overview table at http://www.regionalization.org/ProvChart.html, last updated, June 24, 2003.

Provincial-Territorial Finance Ministers. (2001). *Addressing Fiscal Imbalance*. Victoria, British Columbia.

Provincial-Territorial Ministers of Health. (2000). *Understanding Canada's health care costs: Final report*. Winnipeg, Manitoba.

Rasmussen, K. (2001). Regionalization and collaborative government: A new direction for health system governance. In Adams, D. (Ed.), *Federalism, democracy and health policy in Canada* (pp 239-270). School of Policy Studies, Institute of Intergovernmental Relations, Queen's University, McGill-Queen's University Press.

Redden, C. J. (1999). Rationing health care in the community: Engaging citizens in health care decision making. *Journal of Health Politics, Policy and Law*, 24, 1363-1389.

Regional Health Authorities of Manitoba. (2001, June 12). Regionalization of health services in Manitoba. http://www.rham.mb.ca/about/region.html.

Simpson, J. (1999, May 26). The thrills, the chills of health-care spending. *The Globe and Mail*, p. A14.

Soderstrom, L. (1999 May 14). Department of Economics. McGill University. *Interview*. Montreal, Quebec.

Soderstrom, L. & Bozzini, L. (1994). Public decision-making in public health care systems. In Lemco, J. (Ed.), *National health care: Lessons for the United States and Canada* (pp. 245-273). Ann Arbor, MI: the University of Michigan Press.

Soderstrom, L., Tousignant, P. & Kaufman, T. (1999). The health and cost effects of substituting home care for inpatient acute care: A review of the evidence. *Canadian Medical Association Journal*, 160, 1151-1155.

Spurgeon, D. (2004). Canada's federal and provincial governments reach agreements over health care spending. *British Medical Journal*, 329, 704-705.

Swenden, W. (2002). Asymmetric federalism and coalition-making in Belgium. *Publius: The Journal of Federalism*, 32, 67-87.

Wessen, A. F. (1999). The comparative study of health care reform. In Powell, F. D. & Wessen, A. F. (Eds.), *Health care systems in transition: An international perspective* (pp. 3-24). Thousand Oaks, CA: Sage Publications.

White, G. (2002). Treaty federalism in Northern Canada: Aboriginal-Government Land Claims Boards. *Publius:The Journal of Federalism*, 32, 89-114.

Working Group Synthesis Report. (1997). Striking a balance. In *National Health Forum, Canadian Health Action: Building a Legacy*. Vol. 2 (pp. 26-45). Ottawa, Ontario.

CLSCs in Quebec:
Thirty Years of Community Action

Benoît Gaumer
Marie-Josée Fleury

INTRODUCTION

Local community service centres (CLSCs) grew out of the social transformations in Quebec in the decades of the 1960s and 1970s, the period known as the Quiet Revolution. At that time, this predominantly French, Catholic province in Canada launched a series of major reforms, primarily in the realms of education and health. The watchword for this new, secularized society was "Masters in our own house". This quasi-revolution, unmarked by any real violence, stood out for its climate of popular participation in political life (which was particularly intense), in the form of citizens' committees and the creation of community organizations[1] in poor urban neighbourhoods. This quite exceptional grassroots mobilization was highly prominent in Montreal, Quebec's metropolis. The first citizens' groups appeared in the period from 1963 to 1968. They were essentially pressure groups whose main activity was to lead actions demanding measures to address specific problems of urban life, including health problems (Godbout & Collin, 1977). A number of community or popular medical clinics sprang up in Montreal, such as the Pointe St. Charles Community Clinic and the St. Jacques citizens' clinic (Boivin, 1988).

Parallel to this emergence of autonomous groups inventing new forms of empowerment and control over health and social problems in poor neighbourhoods, the new social affairs minister in Quebec launched a fundamental reform of its healthcare system. Local health centres, later rebaptized local community service centres (CLSCs), were gradually set up, not without some reluctance on the part of the political authorities, and opposition from certain interest groups. They were to be the point of entry into the new health and social service system. These new health organizations emerged in the North American context of developing *Neighbourhood Health Centers* or *Free Clinics* in the United States (Sardell, 1988). On the international front, this movement would later be taken up by the World Health Organization and dubbed primary care. Developing locally, often at the initiative of individuals or groups involved in their community, each CLSC differentiated itself by the dynamics of its community. Gradually, however, these organizations were remodelled under the centralizing efforts of Quebec's department of health and social services (MSSS). Basing themselves on the concept of *comprehensive medicine*, the CLSCs were to transform the healthcare system and lead it away from the medical model that predominated at the time, toward a more social model. Added to these two major roles was the community action component, whose objectives and content would become more specific over time.

To fulfil their medical, social and community functions, a new professional category appeared in the CLSCs alongside physicians, nurses and clinical social workers: community organizers. When the first CLSCs were created, community organizers consisted mainly of highly committed activists in community action–i.e., in mobilization and development. Their place in relation to the other more classic actors–professionals in health care and social services–and the way these community organizers became professionalized are questions of interest to us. Although few in number, the community organizers were to play a particularly important role in developing and supporting community organizations, and the CLSCs emerged as bona fide laboratories for social innovation, especially when they were first created.

In the thirty active years of their existence, the CLSCs went through a number of transition periods that at times altered their orientations considerably. Community action was often the specific orientation that came under challenge. The 1980s were particularly decisive, with pressure from the MSSS forcing the 160 CLSCs to standardize their practice and develop priority areas such as mental health and home care for elderly individuals with reduced autonomy. New legislation on health and social services was passed in 1991, consolidating the role of CLSCs as the basis of the system. The tribulations of these primary care health and social service institutions were nonetheless not over. Increasingly amalgamated with the long-term residential care centres as of 1996, inheriting the heavy burden of the shift to ambulatory care that was beginning at that point, the CLSCs' ability to maintain their threefold mission was increasingly under debate, as was the possibility of the CLSCs having to sacrifice their community action role. With the advent of family medicine groups[2] whose aim is to bring primary care medicine in private clinics and CLSCs closer together, and with the massive restructuring of the system in the form of local service networks including the merger of

CLSCs and hospital centers, the question now is whether the CLSCs will lose their originality definitively.

The CLSCs, with their strengths and weaknesses, thus offer an interesting illustration of the kinds of health promotion initiatives that can be undertaken to influence social determinants of health and illness, starting with our healthcare systems that are all too often centred on the curative and on the individual. In what follows, the first years of the CLSCs' existence will be examined through their functions and mandates. In the 1980s, these organizations were substantially revised, marking a major change in their trajectory. After looking at this period, the role of community organizers (which reflects the original position held by the CLSCs) will be examined. The two other sections will focus on the key roles played by the CLSCs in the emergence of community organizations, in home support services, and in mental health. Finally, the CLSCs' prospects for the future will be discussed in the context of major reforms.

THE CLSCS' MANDATE AND FUNCTIONS: THE FIRST YEARS

The idea of creating public primary healthcare centres in Quebec came from the report by the commission of inquiry into health and welfare (Commission d'enquête sur la santé et le bien-être social–CESBES), filed in 1970, which marked the creation of the Quebec healthcare system. Formed in 1966, the commission was particularly interested in these institutions in its proposals for the general reorganization of the system of health and social services in the province. Highly impressed by the experiments conducted in this area in other countries and particularly in certain American states such as California and New York, it recommended that such structures be set up in Quebec to spearhead the new healthcare system. The commission proposed more of a hierarchy in healthcare services, with three basic levels–general, specialized and ultra-specialized care–corresponding to three levels of organization: the local community service centre (CLSC), the community health centre (CHC) and the university hospital centre (UHC). All would have to incorporate curative, preventive and rehabilitative care. It referred extensively to the Health Insurance Plan of Greater New York and to the Kaiser Foundation, as well as to certain popular clinics known as Neighbourhood Health Centers, to show how these organizations considerably reduced costly reliance on specialized care delivered in the hospitals. Curiously, the commission was not fully knowledgeable as to the existence of popular clinics in Montreal and Quebec City that reflected the same spirit as the American clinics (Gouvernement du Québec, 1970).[3]

Shortly after the commission's report was tabled, the government grouped health services together with social services under the aegis of the new department of social affairs (MAS–Ministère des Affaires sociales), and the minister in charge was the former president of the commission. The minister and his officers immediately began to implement the plan to reorganize health services and social services. This initiative found concrete expression with the passage of the Act respecting health services and social services in December 1971. The commission's local health centre (CLS) was to become the local community service centre (CLSC), incorporating medical care, prevention and social services within one structure, thus concretizing the plan for "comprehensive medicine" that underlay the entire philosophy of the commission's report.

The CLSC was created as an autonomous institution completely independent of the hospitals and social service centres[4], which in turn were newly created. Run by a local board of directors, the CLSCs were 100% financed by the department of social affairs (MAS). Their mandate was to offer a range of basic health care and social services, for the most part delivered by multidisciplinary teams to the local territory's population. This range of services comprised three main categories of services: basic curative and preventive health care, social services to meet the current needs of individuals, and community action aimed at encouraging the population to take part in identifying and solving health and social problems through information and group discussion (MAS, 1972). Community action, with its innovative and often provocative and challenging thrust, would be the subject of criticism and indeed virulent opposition from more conservative circles. The local territory served by the CLSCs was made up of a population of about 10,000 people in rural areas and about 30,000 in urban areas–a dimension considered adequate to achieve the objectives of personalized services and citizen involvement. To cover the province of Quebec, the number of CLSCs required was 200, once the network was completed (Rodriguez, 2003).

In the first two years of the reform–i.e., between 1972 and 1974, sixty-five CLSCs were created in the various regions in the province (Bélanger, 1992). The implementation process consisted of setting up a committee of citizens interested in the territory's health and welfare issues. A number of these committees were set up even before any department representative had instigated training. Once accredited, they received an implementation budget to enable them to hire the necessary resources to analyze the health and social service needs of the population in the territory, proceed with the relevant consultations, and draw up a program in response to these local needs. After the process was completed (which could take a year to a year-and-a-half), the promotion committee would present its program plan to the department. The committee would then negotiate with the department to determine the new CLSC's annual budget. This approach gave rise to considerable diversity in the first CLSC programs, and in their level of financial resources.

An initial implementation assessment was done in 1975, which attested to this diversity and the relatively high importance ascribed to community action, depending on the territory. CLSCs could then be classified in accordance with programs to be adopted, using three models: the model centred on services; the model geared toward community development; and the mixed model. In the model centring on services, the type of practice was characterized by the almost exclusive predominance of curative health services. This type of practice was essentially found in CLSCs in which physicians were remunerated by the act. This was also found in rural, semi-rural or urban areas. In the model centred on community development, community action became a reference point for other professions—medicine, nursing care and social services—with prevention being the predominant interventional approach used both in individual consultations and in groups. The CLSC was considered to be a specific instrument in the community to effect more comprehensive social changes. An anti-service ideology was often found: traditional types of professionalism were criticized and considered to be an obstacle to achieving the objectives deemed most valuable, such as social mobilization and transformation of the community. This type of CLSC nonetheless had more difficulty integrating in the network of health services. In the mixed model, the preventive component was important but preponderance was given to the curative component, with community action reduced to its smallest share. In this model and that of community development, physicians received a salary, like the other professionals (Champoux et al., 1975).

In the second half of the 1970s, the development of new CLSCs slowed down. The government cited difficulties with the budget, and postponed any decision about which model to prioritize. Despite the fact that by 1975, after three years, there were already 70 CLSCs, in the subsequent five years only fifteen new centres were created, all of them in 1976-77.

THE SHIFT IN THE 1980s:
MORE SPECIFIC BUT NARROWER MANDATES

It was not until 1981 that the department of social affairs (MAS) decided to show confidence in the CLSCs with a concrete gesture, entrusting them with specific mandates and responsibilities in distributing services. It officialized its formal intention to cover the entire province of Quebec with a comprehensive, generalized system of public, primary care services in health and social services (MAS, 1987). One hundred and sixty health and social service districts were identified to constitute the geographic framework for these services. While no CLSCs were set up between 1977 and 1981, the 1980-81 fiscal year was marked by the opening of sixteen new establishments. The pace slowed in the following two years, but began accelerating again as of 1983-1984. There no longer appeared to be anything to stop the completion of the network to cover the entire province of Quebec, yet the difficulties characterizing these initial developments did not disappear.

In January 1986, the federation of CLSCs, a vigorous spokesgroup created in 1975, presented a brief to the new minister of health and social services[5] entitled *"Les CLSC face aux enjeux des années 90: une nécessaire consolidation."* This was not only a plea to complete the network, it reiterated the main reasons that slowed the process of setting up these new organizations: challenges both by community groups that did not want to be co-opted and by professional groups that saw their interests threatened. The federation denounced the inequalities in the development of CLSCs–inequalities associated with region, territory and year of operationalization–while all CLSCs had to fulfil the same responsibilities. The aging of the population, mental health and accessibility of services were considered to be priorities requiring further investment. Parallel to this, a departmental committee tabled a report on the CLSCs. It supported the conclusions of the federation of CLSCs that the diversity they displayed in their range of services undermined their efficacy (MSSS, 1987). It recommended that the CLSCs offer a common program consisting of five essential types of services associated with: current health and social services, home support, mental health and the children/family/youth sector. It also suggested that the choice of the final program be based on local priorities. It reaffirmed the need to prioritize the development of primary health care and services as advocated by the World Health Organization, in order to eliminate all obstacles to the accessibility of services.

As soon as the committee's report was tabled, there was an angry outcry on the part of community organizers (Bourque, 1990). The basic range of services defended by the committee was vigorously assailed by those defending the specificity of each CLSC and its roots in the local community. The risk of community work being abandoned or reduced to its smallest component was indeed high, as the committee distinguished between two types of community action: one involving the CLSC's community organizers giving their support to the various in-house programs, and the other involving the responsibility of organizations other than CLSCs, such as those working to curb unemployment or to improve housing.

In 1991, the Quebec government passed a new law on the organization of health and social services that in large measure pushed aside the preceding legislation dating back to 1971. The political will to place the citizen at the centre of the system was affirmed. Decentralization of the healthcare system's management was reinforced, with the creation of eighteen regional health and social services boards; however, this did not mean moving toward genuine regionalization with taxation powers conferred on the new boards. In this new framework, the CLSCs, which had been a marginal component of the health and social services in the early '70s, were becoming a major partner, representing primary care that was increasingly recognized as essential. Some nonetheless continued to fear that such recognition by the central and regional authorities (on which the CLSCs depended almost entirely for their funding) would result into a damaging loss of autonomy. They argued that this would affect their capacity to influence the socio-economic determinants of health such as unemployment, and would sacrifice community action. Community organizers, in particular, who had turned their work into a profession, were gradually imposed as new actors–not without difficulty in certain CLSCs.

COMMUNITY ORGANIZERS: THE ORIGINAL ACTORS

In the first years, the intensity of community action led by the CLSCs varied enormously depending on the CLSC model that was predominant. The same was true of the profile of community organizers. In poor areas where most of the first popular clinics were born, there were many community organizers with a number of years' experience as grassroots organizers. The majority of them had university training–some with a bachelor's degree, a Master's or in some cases, a doctorate. Politically on the Left, defending the poor and working classes, they were often the instigators of the popular mobilization that led to the creation of the first CLSCs. Over the years, young community organizers emerged who were trained in social service in community colleges (CEGEPS)[6] but were inexperienced, and who had difficulty gaining recognition from other professionals such as physicians and nurses. The exception here was social work practitioners, as the work performed by young community organizers was an extension of theirs. These clinical social workers were not very numerous until the mid-1980s when the majority of them in the social service centres that were abolished were transferred into CLSCs. Their arrival in the CLSCs in large numbers would not facilitate consolidation of the profession of community organizer, particularly since the department put off recruiting these new professionals, seeking instead to limit their numbers and their qualifications (Alary & Leseman, 1975). As one social worker indicated at the time, it was sometimes difficult to distinguish clinical social workers from other psycho-social practitioners, especially community organizers, when they used the same approach and working methods—i.e., focusing action on groups rather than on casework.

Physicians and nurses, on the other hand, were clearly distinguished by their training and the type of medical services they offered the population. General practitioners who chose to work in CLSCs did so out of a sense of conviction, and had to face opposition (especially in the early years), if not a boycott of the CLSCs by the Quebec federation of general practitioners (Fédération des FMOQ)[7] and the majority of the medical corps, outraged by the clearly progressive political orientation of the first such centres. Nurses, for the most part, came from the former county health units,[8] essentially delivering preventive medical services such as vaccinations or monitoring the health of pregnant women or newborns. They had little contact with clinical social workers, and community action was not part of their tradition. Less politically involved, they observed with cautious detachment their new professional partners' efforts to mobilize the population. Their attention was directed more toward the development of interdisciplinary work, with physicians and clinical social workers (D'Amour, 2001).

The development of an organizational culture that was common to practitioners or professionals in CLSCs was laborious, and all the more so in that for a long time the community organizers refused all professionalism, preferring to draw their expertise from hands-on work in the field (Poupart et al., 1986). Through their affiliation with a province-wide union (Confédération des syndicats nationaux–CSN), as of

1976 they had in fact negotiated a definition of their professional practice with their employer, the department of social affairs (MAS). This definition was based on three functions: "identifying and analyzing the needs of the population with the groups concerned; . . . designing, coordinating and actualizing community organization programs to meet the needs of the community and promote its development; and acting as a resource person for the groups" (Lachapelle, 2003, p. 18).

In 1988, community organizers preferred to be called community practitioners, and created the *Regroupement québécois des intervenantes et intervenants en action communautaire* (RQIIAC)[9] to represent them. Although some still wanted to avoid all forms of professionalism, the idea was nonetheless to consolidate a new profession. Finding it at times difficult to demarcate themselves from clinical social workers, who had been represented for a long time by a professional order, their expertise, confirmed by experience in the field, led them to use one of the three major modes of social work almost exclusively: community action or organization. The two other modes of social work–individual psychosocial intervention and group intervention–were instead reserved for clinical social workers (Lachapelle, 2003). Often opposed to traditional practitioners of social work (whom they saw as professional agents of social integration), in the early years, community organizers were first and foremost activists–agents of social change. Over time, this way of being and this profile of intervention for community practitioners changed and became professionalized. They were seen for a long time as the "enfant terrible" of the CLSC, and their relations were fairly strained with the executive administration, which was increasingly preoccupied with planning and administering in-house services. With the years, an alliance was nonetheless forged, with most CLSCs seeing themselves as "an important community lever in local communities that are attempting to organize themselves" (Favreau & Hurtubise, 1992).

CLSCS:
A LABORATORY FOR COMMUNITY ORGANIZATIONS

In Quebec in 2004, more than twelve thousand community groups linked together on a sectoral basis (e.g., mental health, home support for the elderly) with mandates that were primarily local but also sub-regional or regional, employed more than 150,000 people (Lachapelle, 2003). Nearly 4,000 of them were in large part funded by the department of health and social services (MSSS). Numerous community organizations (whose figures could not be estimated due to the fragmentary nature of the available studies) developed at the initiative of the CLSCs or benefited from their technical (if not financial) support through grants from the department. The CLSCs often acted as spokesgroups for the community groups, and played a role in getting the Quebec government to gradually recognize autonomous community organizations that were committed to community action. Relations were not always harmonious between CLSCs, on one hand, which were entirely funded by the department and were under pressure to standardize their operations, and community organizations on the other, which were partially funded by the department through regional health and social services boards[10] but jealously guarded their autonomy. Some CLSCs operating along the lines of the service-based model strictly focused on the MSSS' programs and used few community organizers, given their tendency to transfer part of their services to community organizations. Others that were closer to the model advocating community development were characterized by a close alliance between the executive administration, community practitioners and community organizations, and attached greater importance to partnering initiatives centring on social prevention and community development. A third category, the mixed model, was midway between the other two: the executive administration and community organizers oscillated between a limited social commitment and their responsibilities as public employees, representing and dependent on the MSSS (Favreau & Hurtubise, 1993).

Community organizations were to play an important role in the shift toward ambulatory care in Quebec's healthcare system. Drastic cutbacks in the mid-'90s, accompanied by hospital closures, led the MSSS to increasingly support the private non-profit voluntary sector, which allowed the government to withdraw without cutting back too far in health and social services for the population. This reliance on community organizations, which it subsidized more or less sparingly, was particularly used by the MSSS to implement its policy on mental health. The mandate it gave to the CLSCs from their inception was to develop home support services, essentially for elderly citizens with reduced autonomy. This illustrates the reliance on community action that gradually encompassed the CLSC professionals as a whole, rather than just the community practitioners.

ESSENTIAL SERVICES:
HOME SUPPORT AND MENTAL HEALTH

It was with the development of home support programs that community action began to take a detour, essentially via the community practitioners on the CLSC's multidisciplinary team. In this process, community practitioners played a pivotal role, questioning practices and favouring teamwork and co-ordination for the CLSC with other institutional and community resources. In the area of home support, where public funding is not on a par with needs, the CLSC was most often called upon to develop new services by stimulating local initiatives: in transportation, food, sitting services (for the elderly), support groups, etc. The first mandate–home support services–that the MSSS conferred on the CLSCs in the midst of a crisis over recognition allowed the CLSCs to build on their credibility and allowed the community organizers in particular to demonstrate their ability to develop intersectoral collaboration. In 2005, MSSS home support policy still essentially depended on the CLSCs integrated in the new local service networks (CLSCs, residential long-term care centres and general and specialized hospital centres), in partnership with a mosaic of community organizations. After witnessing accelerated growth for nearly ten years now, the policy will have to be maintained because of the aging population and the shift toward ambulatory care, and the deinstitutionalization and non-institutionalization of elderly people, handicapped people and clientele with severe mental health problems (MSSS, 2003). There will be a call for the development of home support for vulnerable clienteles such as these, through further mobilization of the local communities.

The CLSCs have also played an important role in mental health. Managing mental health disorders is a major public health issue, and the prevalence of such disorders in the population is estimated at about 20% (Health Canada, 2002). In Canada, the annual or lifelong prevalence for major depression is between 5% and 8-10%, and for anxiety disorders, between 12% and 21% (MSSS, 2005). In Quebec, the CLSCs are the only suppliers of public services to offer current psycho-social services to an adult clientele. For young people (0-18 years), the CLSCs offer primary care and basic services. For the past few years, they have also been offering specialized services for the clientele with severe mental health problems, which represents between 2% and 3% of the population. The services offered are primarily related to clientele follow-up in the community, which is of varying intensity depending on the needs. In developing and supporting community groups in mental health that represent nearly one third of the organizations financed by the department of health and social services (MSSS), the CLSCs have played a particularly important role. Given the importance of the field of mental health and the rise in the number of people with reduced autonomy, the CLSCs represent an indispensable actor in the healthcare system in Quebec.

FUTURE PROSPECTS

In 2004-2005, the CLSCs lost their autonomy, which was marked by the presence of an autonomous board of directors made up of local elected representatives. The new law passed by Quebec's National Assembly reorganized the public network of health and social services on a new territorial basis, comprising 95 local service networks grouped into 18 health and social service regions. In each of the local territories, the CLSCs, residential long-term care centres, and general and specialized hospital centres were merged and must co-ordinate their service delivery with other suppliers in the territory: private medical offices, community organizations, etc. The local service networks are aimed at improving the integration of health care and social services, the consistency and quality of the services provided (e.g., accessibility, continuity, no duplication of care). The earlier period of the CLSCs with the residential long-term care centres, involved in the neighbourhood in the mid-1990s, had already played a part in standardizing the CLSCs' program of activities and diluting their community action. From now on, given that the CLSCs have been merged with formidable organizations like hospital centres with a primarily curative vision of health, what will become of social and community action, and initiatives aimed at prevention and the promotion of health? How are community practitioners going to reposition themselves in relation to a new executive administration that is more remote than the former administration of the CLSCs and their local grassroots?

Some indications are fairly reassuring, such as the appointment of former CLSC directors who have supported community action thus far, at the head of new local coalitions. The local networks have also been given responsibility toward the full spectrum of their population's health in their respective territory, which specifically leads them to integrate the expertise developed by the CLSCs and their community practitioners: identification of the populations' needs, prevention and health promotion, consideration of the continuum of essential care offered to

vulnerable clientele, co-ordination of services, etc. Currently generalized to include all care providers, the process of activating integrated
service networks began more than a decade ago (Fleury, 2005). The first
networks took shape around specific clientele or health problems: severe mental health disorders, the elderly clientele with reduced autonomy, Type 2 diabetes, etc. The CLSCs have played a central role in
establishing and co-ordinating these networks. In the context of these
reforms, their services were often consolidated, as well. The same was
true for the creation of family medicine groups, for which one of the key
orientations was to reinforce and better co-ordinate the CLSCs' psycho-
social activities with curative care. It is conceivable, then, that in this
process of generalizing integrated service networks in Quebec, the
CLSCs may strengthen their social, community and prevention/promo-
tion roles and action.

CONCLUSION

The CLSC movement in Quebec, despite its difficulties, weaknesses
and uncertain future, offers a good illustration of a participatory program integrating health and social services. This movement, at the outset, was not an isolated one in North America. We find it almost
simultaneously in the United States and a number of Canadian provinces. For Quebec, they were deemed to be "a very important social
movement (which) propelled that province into the forefront in the area
of community health" (Wood, 1986). Born in the creative enthusiasm of
the local communities, the CLSCs deliberately aimed at mobilizing local communities and encouraging their empowerment in taking greater
control over their own health and welfare.

In the last thirty years, the CLSCs went through a number of crises
that verged on challenging their legitimacy and indeed their very existence. The three main functions attributed to the CLSCs at the outset
were medical, social and community care and services, stemming from
popular initiatives and the political will shown (although not always ex-
plicitly) by the department of social affairs (MAS) in the early 1970s.
Community action represented the highly original dimension of "medico-
socio-community" actions developed by the 160 CLSCs or health centres that encompassed the overall territory of Quebec until the current
reform.

The "spontaneism" of the first wave of CLSCs, based on the model of
community clinics or "free clinics" in the United States, inspired fear

among certain groups of professionals such as physicians, who took part in this movement in very small numbers only. It also provoked reserve among the politicians at the time such as those in the Parti Québécois, despite their social democratic leanings. This explains the CLSCs' long gestation period. The province of Quebec was not fully covered by CLSCs until 1989, after the MSSS succeeded in bringing them in step by imposing common programs whose content–and financing–were almost entirely under its control. To date, their threefold mission (medical, social and community) remains, despite the restructuring and loss of autonomy of these institutions. Community practitioners, like the community organizations that are one of their main partners, are still there and still highly active. The public-private partnerships now being advocated by the current government of Quebec could not manage without the CLSCs' expertise, which has succeeded in resisting numerous crises and challenges.

NOTES

1. One section of this article focuses on community organizations. They are generally small, non-profit resources whose mandates are limited to one or several programs (e.g., self-help groups for peers or family members, crisis centres, suicide prevention centres).

2. Aside from the CLSCs, there are private clinics in Quebec that group together the vast majority of general practitioners and family physicians. To co-ordinate these two types of organizations that deliver primary health care, groups of family physicians are being set up throughout the province.

3. This oversight was probably deliberate, as the commission's socio-political makeup and its official mandate did not allow it to associate with these popular movements that were contesting the established order or were part of the radical Left.

4. The social service centres were created in the wake of the reform in the early 1970s, on a regional and sub-regional basis. They were eliminated with the new reform at the beginning of the 1990s, after the largest segment of their clinical social workers was cut and transferred to CLSCs.

5. In 1986, the department of social affairs (MAS) changed its name to the department of health and social services (MSSS), after surrendering its income security responsibilities to another department.

6. CEGEPs, otherwise known as *Collèges d'enseignement général et professionnel*, are educational institutions that were created in the educational reform in the late 1960s. They are an intermediary level between comprehensive high schools and universities, preparing students for university as well as developing short-term cycles of vocational training.

7. The *Fédération des médecins omnipraticiens du Québec* is the only professional association representing practically all general practitioners in the province, and was founded in Quebec City on January 12, 1962 (*Le Médecin du Québec*, Vol. 1, No. 1, June

1965, p. 21). Specialists are represented by the *Fédération des médecins spécialistes*, which is much more traditional in its professional demands.

8. The county health units, set up along the American model as of 1926, covered the entire territory of Quebec until the CLSCs were created. As basic public health units, they offered prevention services exclusively.

9. See the RQIIAC's web site, www.rqiiac.qc.ca, which is well-documented and up-dated. In January 2003, the number of community organizers' positions in the CLSCs was estimated at 400.

10. In 1991, 18 regional health and social services boards (RRSSS) replaced the 12 regional health and social services councils (CRSSS) that had been created in 1972, at the same time as the CLSCs and the social service centres. The CRSSS and the RRSSS were regional decentralizing structures associated with the department of social affairs (MAS), which became the department of health and social services (MSSS) in 1986.

REFERENCES

Alary, J. & Leseman, F. (1975). *Les CLSC, Étude des dimensions sociales et communautaires*, Rapport au MAS, Montréal.

Béland, F. (1998). *Preventive and Primary Care Access Systems: CLSCs as Neighborhood and Social Service Centers in Quebec*, In Health Care Systems in Transition. An International Perspective. F.D. Powell & A.F. Wessen (eds). Thousand Oaks, CA : SAGE Publications Inc., 173-198.

Bélanger, J.P. (1992). *Le développement des soins primaires au Québec: le cas des CLSC*, Colloque international sur les soins de santé primaires, Montréal.

Boivin, R. (1988). *Histoire de la clinique des citoyens de St-Jacques*, VLB éditeur, Montréal.

Bourque, D. (1990). "Les CLSC à la croisée des chemins. La mise au pas tranquille des CLSC," *Nouvelles pratiques sociales*, *3*, (2) 43-57.

Bozzini, L. (1988). "Local Community Services Centers (CLSCs) in Quebec: Description, Evaluation, Perspectives, *Journal of Public Health Policy*, *9*, 346-375.

Brunet, J. (1972), *Politique en matière de santé du MAS*, Document de travail, MAS, Québec.

Champoux, L. et al. (1975). *Rapport du groupe d'étude sur le fonctionnement des CLSC dit "Rapport bilan"*, Rapport au MAS, Montréal.

D'Amour, D. (2001). "Collaboration entre les infirmières et les médecins de famille. Pourquoi et dans quelles conditions?" *Ruptures*, *8*, 1, 136-145.

Desrosiers, G. & B. Gaumer (1987). *L'occupation d'une partie du champ des soins de première ligne par l'hôpital général: faits, conséquences, alternatives*, Rapport présenté à la Commission d'enquête sur les services de santé et de services sociaux, Les publications du Québec, Québec.

Favreau, L. & Y. Hurtubise (1993). *CLSC et communautés locales La contribution de l'organisation communautaire*, Les Presses de l'Université du Québec, Sainte-Foy.

Favreau, L., R. Lachapelle & L. Chagnon (dir) (1994). *Pratiques d'action communautaire en CLSC Acquis et défis d'aujourd'hui*, Les Presses de l'Université du Québec, Ste-Foy.

Fédération des CLSC du Québec (1977). *Rôles et fonctions des CLSC*, texte rédigé conjointement avec le MAS.

Fédération des CLSC du Québec (janvier 1983). *Le développement de "services sociaux locaux": un nouveau mode d'organisation du système de distribution des services*, mémoire remis à Monsieur Pierre-Marc Johnson, ministre des Affaires sociales du Québec.

Fédération des CLSC (janvier 1986). *Les CLSC face aux enjeux des années 90: une nécessaire consolidation*, mémoire remis à Madame Thérèse Lavoix-Roux, ministre de la Santé et des Services sociaux.

Fleury, M.-J. (2005). "Models of Integrated Service Networks and Key Conditions for their Operationalization," *International Journal of Integrated Care*, 5: April-June 2005, 1-17.

Gaumer, B. & G. Desrosiers (2004). "L'histoire des CLSC au Québec: reflet des contradictions et des luttes à l'intérieur du Réseau," *Ruptures*, *10*, 1, 52-70.

Godbout, J. T. & J. Guay (1989). *Le communautaire public le cas d'un CLSC*, études et documents no 62, INRS Urbanisation, Montréal.

Godbout, J. & J. P. Collin, (1977). *Les organismes populaires en milieu urbain: contrepouvoir ou nouvelle pratique professionnelle?* Rapport de recherche no. 3, INRS Urbanisation, Montréal.

Godbout, J. & N. Martin (1974). *Participation et Innovation, L'implantation des centres locaux de services communautaires et les organismes communautaires autonomes*, recherche conjointe ENAP et INRS Urbanisation, Université du Québec, Montréal.

Gouvernement du Québec (2000). *Rapport et recommandations de la Commission d'étude sur les services de santé et de services sociaux*. Les solutions émergentes, Publications du Québec, Québec.

Gouvernement du Québec (1988). *Rapport de la Commission d'enquête sur les services de santé et de services sociaux*, Publications du Québec, Québec.

Gouvernement du Québec (1970). *Rapport de la Commission d'enquête sur la santé et le bien-être social, deuxième partie, titre deuxième, le Régime de santé, tome II, la santé*, Publications du Québec, Québec.

Lachapelle, R. (dir.) (2003). *L'organisation communautaire en CLSC Cadre de référence et pratiques*, Les Presses de l'Université Laval, Québec.

Ministère de la Santé et des Services sociaux (2003). *Chez soi: le premier choix. La politique de soutien à domicile*, www.msss.gouv.qc.ca.

Ministère de la Santé et des Services sociaux (MSSS) (1987). *Rapport du comité de réflexion et d'analyse des services dispensés par les CLSC* (Rapport Brunet), Gouvernement du Québec, Direction de la planification et de l'évaluation et Direction générale de la prévention et des services communautaires, Québec.

Ministère des Affaires sociales (MAS) (1972). *Les Centres locaux de services communautaires*, Gouvernement du Québec, Québec.

Ministère de la Santé et des Services sociaux (MSSS) (2005), Plan d'action en santé mentale 2005-2008, Gouvernement du Québec, Québec.

Parenteau, F. (1986). *Historique, actualité et avenir des CLSC*, Mémoire présenté à la Commission d'enquête sur les services de santé et de services sociaux par la Direction des services communautaires du ministère de la Santé et des Services sociaux, Québec.

Poupart, R., et al. (1986). *La création d'une culture organisationnelle: le cas des CLSC*, Centre de recherche en gestion de l'Université du Québec et Fédération des CLSC.

Renaud, G. (1978). *L'éclatement de la profession en service social*. Montréal, Éditions coopératives Albert Saint Martin.

Robichaud, J. B. & C. Quiviger, (1991), *Active Communities. A Study of Local Community Health and Social Service Centres in Canada in 1988*, The Canadian Council on Social Development, Ottawa.

Rodriguez, C. (2003). "Scénarios d'intégration: le cas des CLSC urbains, une mission impossible? Ruptures, *9*, (2), 92-109.

Roy, M. (1987). *Les CLSC ce qu'il faut savoir*, Éditions Saint-Martin, Montréal.

Sardell, A. (1988). *The U.S. Experiment in Social Medecine The Community Health Center Program, 1965-1986*. University of Pittsburgh Press, Pittsburgh.

Taylor, S. H. & R.W. Roberts, (1985). *Theory and Practice of Community Social Work*, Columbia University Press, New York.

Wood, J. E. (1986). *Hygeia vs Panakeia: The Community Health Centre in Canada*, thesis for the degree of master of arts, department of sociology and anthropology, Carleton University, Ottawa.

Feminist Health Care in a Hostile Environment: A Case Study of the Womancare Health Center

Cheryl A. Hyde

INTRODUCTION

During the last several decades, health policies and programs have undergone extensive changes in the United States. One of the most significant developments during this time has been the recognition of, and responses to, women's health needs. Even though gender inequities in health care remain, the current situation is far different from the 1960s, when women's health concerns were barely acknowledged as "real" (Geary, 1995; Gelb & Palley, 1996; Kraynak, 1994; Morgen, 2002; Nichols, 2000; Rosser, 2002; Ruzek, 1978, 2004; Weisman, 1998; Zimmerman & Hill, 2000). Much of the change in women's health care was, and still is, the result of efforts by the feminist health movement.

This article focuses on some of the accomplishments of, and challenges to, the feminist health movement as exemplified by the experiences in one feminist health center. The story of the Womancare Health Center is noteworthy not only because of its ability to integrate politics and service and its array of programs, but also because it successfully negotiated the challenges presented by a politically hostile environment. The case study of this organization underscores the extensive measures undertaken by members of the feminist health movement to continue the work of providing health care to women.

OVERVIEW OF THE FEMINIST HEALTH MOVEMENT

Feminists, according to anthropologist Sandra Morgen, "view the health care system of the United States as a microcosm that reflects the sexism and economic injustices of the larger society" (1990, p. 9; see also Nichols, 2000; Weisman, 1998; Zimmerman & Hill, 2000). The quest for reproductive choice is the essence of the feminist health movement and the concept of "self-help" its primary value (Morgen, 2002; Ruzek, 1978, 1998; Weisman, 1998). The movement's premise is that women can not be free without control over their own bodies, as manifested through egalitarian relationships between care giver and consumer; the promotion of education, self-care, and self-help; and preventative, holistic and natural approaches to medicine (Dixon-Miller, 1993). Key issues include access to contraceptive and abortion services, pre- and post-natal care, HIV/AIDS treatment, workplace health and safety, body image, domestic violence, and mental health. A 1978 brochure by

the Reproductive Rights National Network delineated the main principles of the movement, all of which remain current:

    I. The right to sexual freedom . . .
    II. The right to abstain from parenting . . .
    III. The right to safe, effective and well-understood contraception . . .
    IV. The right to abortion . . .
    V. The right to be free from forced sterilization . . .
    VI. The right to pregnancy disability payments . . .
    VII. Control of the birthing process . . .
    VIII. The right to a safe workplace . . .
    IX. The right to free, quality childcare . . .
    X. The right to quality free medical care . . .
    XI. The right to education about our bodies . . .
    XII. The right to a guaranteed adequate job or income (Reproductive
    Rights National Network, 1978)

The feminist health movement challenges and provides alternatives to
traditional medicine through clinics, educational and self-help associa-
tions, and advocacy groups.

    While women have been healers throughout history (and were perse-
cuted or executed for these activities), the contemporary feminist health
movement generally is seen as beginning in 1971 (Ehrenreich & English,
1979; Morgen, 2002; Ruzek, 1978; Weisman, 1998). In the fall of that
year, Carol Downer, a Los Angeles abortion rights activist, "appropri-
ated" a speculum from a gynecologist's office and brought together a
group of women to learn about their own and each other's reproductive
anatomies. With abortion illegal in many states, these women quickly
realized that knowledge about one's own body offered the possibility of
alternative, natural and woman-controlled health care (including abortions and birth control). The mystique of the gynecologist' office could be
contested. Health cooperatives formed in the area and members began
charting fertility cycles, offering self-exams, preparing home remedies,
and performing menstrual extractions. The Los Angeles Feminist Women's
Health Center opened and provided classes to women in the area and
across the country in self-help, serving as a prototype for many feminist
health centers founded during the 1970s. By the end of the decade there
was over 100 clinics and an estimated 1,200 self-help health groups
(Nichols, 2000; Weisman, 1998).

    Educational and political action groups also formed to address women's
health needs. Perhaps most well-known is the Boston Women's Health

Book Collective, which published the best selling *Our Bodies, Ourselves* in 1970 (now in its 8th edition and translated into 19 languages). The result of a group of women meeting to discuss health concerns and then circulating research findings that addressed their questions, this book was and is considered "the resource" in women's health. Proceeds from its sale support a women's information and referral organization, as well as various women's health initiatives.

Other significant feminist health organizations started during the 1970s included the Coalition for the Medical Rights for Women (demanded tighter regulations and labeling for drugs and medical devices especially birth control), the National Women's Health Network (worked primarily on federal health policies as related to women's issues), the Reproductive Rights National Network (advocated for reproductive and sexual freedom), the National Abortion Rights Action League (originally founded in 1969 as the National Association for Repeal of Abortion Laws), and DES Action. In the 1980s, the National Black Women's Health Project and the National Latina Health Organization were founded, as were national coalitions that advocated for the health rights of lesbians and women with disabilities (Geary, 1995; Morgen, 2002; Nichols, 2000; Weisman, 1998). Groups, such as the National Organization for Women (NOW), formed taskforces that focused specifically on reproductive rights. Myriad state and regional alliances and community organizations also were founded during the 1970s and 1980s. Across the country, through demonstrations, public hearings, and acts of civil disobedience, women organized for access to safe and legal birth control and abortion services (Morgen, 2002; Ruzek, 1978; Weisman, 1998).

There is little question, however, that the 1973 Roe v. Wade Supreme Court decision, which legalized abortion nationally, was a catalytic moment for the feminist health movement (Gelb & Palley, 1996; Weisman, 1998). Previously illegal activities were now permissible. Yet the decision also galvanized the opposition. From the end of the 1970s and onward, feminists found themselves fighting for, and often losing, their recently acquired gains. With the rise to power of the New Right in the late 1970s, access to safe abortion, specifically, and reproductive care, in general, has been threatened and curtailed.

The New Right, specifically fundamentalist Christian Conservatives, found allies in the Reagan and Bush administrations of the 1980s, and more recently in the current Bush presidency, as well as in Congress. The New Right exhibited three broad strategic trends in its anti-feminist efforts: legislative, fiscal and direct actions (Hyde, 1995). Legislative initiatives focused on regulating sexuality, specifically abortion and reproductive health services, and included ending federal funding for abortion, promoting parental and spousal consent laws, banning sex education programs, supporting conservative politicians and aggressively targeting of pro-choice candidates. Fiscal measures involved cutbacks in or elimination of a number of programs such as Comprehensive Employ- ment Training Act (CETA), which often paid for staff, and Title X (fam- ily planning) grants on which feminist organizations, including health centers, relied. There also were severe reductions in funding sources that supported reproductive health services for low-income women. Grant restrictions were imposed so that organizations that "endorsed" or "promoted" lesbianism, abortion or sex education would not be eligi- ble for federal funds (Dailard, 2001; Gelb & Palley, 1996; Kolk, 1996; Morgen, 2002; Weisman, 1998).

The New Right, however, is perhaps most (in)famous for its direct action protests. Various New Right organizations targeted feminist health clinics and groups through pickets, demonstrations, vandalism, patient intimidation, staff threats, clinic invasions, assaults and bomb- ings. One of the most well-organized anti-abortion campaigns was Op- eration Rescue, led by Joseph Scheidler (Morgen, 2002). His book, *Closed: 99 Ways to Stop Abortion* (Scheidler, 1985), remains the "bi- ble" for anti-abortion activists, as he instructs them in strategies such as the use of bullhorns, the presentation of graphic material for greatest media impact, the picketing of clinic doctor's homes, and the use of pri- vate detectives to find abortion clinic patients and then visiting her and her family. In an indication of the ties that anti-abortion activists had with the White House and Congress, few clinic attacks were investi- gated by the Justice Department during the 1980s.

Given the rise and coalescence of the New Right, recent develop- ments in the feminist health movement largely focused on preserving existing reproductive rights and on countering right wing activism. Ac- tivities included testifying against restrictive legislative measures, clinic defenses such as patient escorts and counter sit-ins, lawsuits against right to life organizations, and marches and rallies. Women's rights or- ganizations, such as NOW and the Feminist Majority Fund, provided detailed accounts of New Right actions to curtail reproductive rights, including clinic bombings, wounding and murder of abortion providers, and most recently, anthrax threats against abortion/family planning clinics (for examples see Bennett-Haigney, 1999; Lonsway, Jackman, Koenig, Leader, & Campos, 2003; National Organization for Women, 2004; Phillips, 1996; Weinstein & Clark, 1998). As a way of broadening its scope, the feminist health movement broadened its focus by addressing sterilization abuse, sexually transmitted diseases, special health needs for lesbians, the elderly, minority and poor women, and AIDs education and counseling (Boston Women's Health Book Collective, 2005; Geary, 1995; Morgen, 2002; Sherwin, 1998; Weisman, 1998).

Detailing the effects of the feminist health movement on the larger U.S. health care system and health policy is beyond the scope of this article (see Baird, 1998; Geary, 1995; Gelb & Palley, 1996; Kraynak, 1994; Palley & Palley, 2000; Ratcliff, 2002; Rosser, 2002; Ruzek, 1998; Weisman, 1998), though there is little doubt that the movement has had a profound impact on the ways in which women now access health care. Many of the changes involved the pressuring of mainstream medical training, practice and research institutions becoming more sensitive to and knowledgeable of the often unique needs and conditions of women and girls. Another set of changes focuses on the enactment of policies and funding acts designed to address women's health concerns. And because the women's health movement is essentially based on consumer empowerment, its activities serve as models for other medically disenfranchised groups (Zimmerman & Hill, 2000). Yet the dominant story of the feminist health movement is its ability to transform itself in order to survive.

CASE STUDY: WOMANCARE HEALTH CENTER

The backbone of the feminist health movement is a network of local-level, independent feminist health clinics. Such an organization may be classified as a social movement agency because its "explicit pursuit of social change is accomplished through the delivery of services" and it has "an ideational duality that encompasses both social movement and human services orientations" (Hyde, 1992, p. 122). Feminist health centers were designed by women as "alternatives to mainstream health care" (Weisman, Curbow, & Khoury, 1995, p. 103). As with the broader feminist health movement, these clinics espoused a mission of self-help, empowerment and collective action; these principles were operationalized in service delivery and governance mechanisms (Morgen, 2002; Ruzek, 1978; Weisman, 1998). While women's health clinics increased during the 1980s and 1990s, many of these were developed by hospitals and did not necessarily share the ideological commitment of the original cohort of feminist health centers (Lundy & Mason, 1994; Weisman, Curbow, & Khoury, 1995). Indeed, few feminist centers from the 1970s remain functioning as independent organizations, having closed or been absorbed by more mainstream institutions (Morgen, 2002).

One clinic that did survive is the Womancare Health Center.[1] Located in the southern United States, the Womancare Health Center was founded in the late 1970s as a self-help support group for women. Since that time, it has developed into a comprehensive women's medical center, though its original mission remains true today: "to empower women through service, education and advocacy, by . . . providing quality gynecological health care, . . . promoting informed decision-making and participatory health care, . . . and advancing women's health and choices through both community and political advocacy" (brochure). This clinic also has the dubious distinction of being among the first targeted by Operation Rescue. Throughout much of the 1980s and into the 1990s, Womancare staff, volunteers and patients were subjected to various forms of intimidation and harassment. Figure 1 presents the New Right threats and the responses by Womancare. Examining how this clinic survived and continued its mission, provides a greater understanding of the feminist health movement's efforts to ensure women's health rights and services in a contentious environment.

Founding Period

As with most feminist health clinics, Womancare emphasized a self-help approach to health care. At its opening in 1977, the staff wrote an open letter to the community and articulated this vision:

FIGURE 1. New Right Actions and the Womancare Health Center

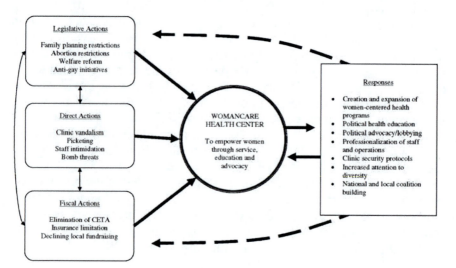

These are the major goals of the women who work at Womancare:
to take back control of our bodies through spreading Self Help . . .
[and] to end oppression of women and all people.

Because self-help is a consumer-centered philosophy, it combined the
principles of consciousness raising, empowerment and education. Usually,
there was a group component to the self-help sessions. Staff, referred to
as "lay health workers," demystified language in their discussions of
medical problems, designed patient advocacy systems, and offered preventative and holistic treatments when possible.

This self-help approach was a key component of a broader, radical
philosophy that guided the center and connected it to larger social
change efforts:

Above all, we have a feminist political commitment. We take ourselves seriously, are anti-imperialistic and anti-capitalistic (1980
Annual Report).

As ways of pursuing this commitment to social change, staff undertook
collections for medical supplies for third world clinics, went on "self-
help" tours across the country, and held community educational programs on feminist health issues. Womancare became a member of a national federation of feminist health care organizations in 1980 in order
to more effectively promote reproductive rights nationally.

This collective, self-help approach also informed internal structures
and processes. Womancare operated with minimal hierarchy and division of labor. Member participation in all aspects of the organization
was emphasized. Jobs were rotated and decisions were reached by consensus. The goal was that each Womancare member would exercise a
strong commitment to the functioning of the clinic, and at the same
time, feel a deep sense of belonging and ownership. Such expectations
were common among feminist health centers during this time.

New Right Actions

Organizations and groups affiliated with the New Right's collective
agenda engaged in various legislative, fiscal and direct action strategies
aimed at impeding, and if possible closing, the Womancare Center.
Legislative and fiscal efforts occurred on national and state levels. The
federal ban on Medicare funds for abortions (Hyde Amendment), restrictions in Family Planning monies, and the elimination of the CETA

program affected the Center's revenue stream, and consequently its service provision and staffing. The state in which Womancare is located, passed parental notification legislation concerning minors obtaining birth control and abortion services (minors must have the written approval of a parent or guardian). The state legislature also attempted to pass spousal notification for abortion and anti-gay initiatives. In 1986, Womancare's malpractice insurance was cancelled without notice (a frequent occurrence for feminist health centers), which endangered its ability to offer various gynecological services. New insurance coverage was obtained, yet with much higher policy premiums. As the 1980s progressed, clinic staff reported a decline in local fundraising. Insurance and funding concerns were linked directly with New Right protest actions.

As noted above, Womancare was one of the original targets of Operation Rescue's national direct action campaign to close down abortion providers. The specific actions of this organization, as well as other anti-abortion mobilizations, created a high-risk environment for center members and patients. At the height of these activities, approximately 500 picketers harassed and intimidated anyone who attempted to enter the clinic. A clinic worker described the experience:

> This morning as I drove up to the health center I could see picketers on the sidewalk. I pulled my car into the staff parking space. I had my two children with me in the care. The picketers stopped walking and just stood behind my car. They were chanting "Stop the killing now." My daughter, who is two, told me she was afraid to get out of the car. I got out and asked the Sergeant if he would carry my daughter in so I could carry in my baby. I felt it was necessary for someone to hold my two year old even though she can walk because she felt afraid and I felt afraid. As I was carrying my baby in a man shouted "Why don't you kill him?" Every week a picketer says something like that to me and my children. It is really affecting me. I find myself dreading going to work on Saturdays and reluctant to bring my children to one of the few places of business that actually offers day care to its employees.

Anti-abortion protesters would inundate the appointment phone line (several hundred phone calls a day), preventing patients from making appointments. Center staff also reported bomb threats that necessitated the closing of the clinic, repeated acts of vandalism (i.e., blood-like substance smeared on center doors, graffiti), and several attempts at clinic invasions by protesters.

In the late 1980s, the Womancare Board of Directors conducted an environmental risk assessment, which delineates their concerns regarding New Right actions:

1. No insurance available–a malpractice.
2. No insurance available for building–liability insurance.
3. Damage to the building from arson, bomb or vandalism resulting in Womancare becoming unable to operate due to building damage, being shut for a prolonged period of time while finding a new location or repairing the present site.
4. Abortion made illegal by the U.S. Supreme Court.
5. Abortion greatly restricted by U.S. Supreme Court.
6. Abortion becomes a state's right issue where [the state] can define the status of abortion in the state and [the state] decides to outlaw or greatly restrict abortion.
7. The clinic loses its non-profit status due to anti-abortion amendments prohibiting tax exempt status for agencies providing abortions
8. Business decreases due to restrictions placed on abortion access–parental or spousal consent, waiting periods, gestational cutback, etc.
9. Business decreases or extraordinary legal fees due to picketing.
10. A serious or fatal complication with bad media relations, results in severe loss of clientele.

This assessment was based not only on what was occurring in the immediate environment, but also on Womancare members' knowledge of the spreading violence against reproductive health centers across the country (Bader & Baird-Windle, 2001; Feldt, 2004; Feminist Women's Health Center, 2000; Morgen, 2002; Ruzek, 1998).

New Right direct actions abated somewhat during the 1990s, in that 500 protesters no longer showed up for several weeks at a time. Nonetheless, staff and patients were still harassed and picketers always were present on the anniversary of *Roe v. Wade*. Womancare also continued to deal with the effects of financial and legislative efforts. Nationally, the *Contract with America* (Gillespie, Gingrich, Schellhas, & Armey, 1994) contained a number of provisions, including measures that foreshadowed the 1996 Defense of Marriage Act, that were antithetical to the mission and goals of Womancare. Many state and local initiatives paralleled terms of the Contract; there was a constant stream of state legislation that sought to end or severely curtail abortion, birth control for minors, sex education, and HIV/AIDS prevention. Federal and state welfare reform initiatives of the mid-1990s had a negative impact in that Center revenues needed to be shifted so that low income women could obtain health care through sliding scales. Not all New Right efforts succeeded, but each necessitated a response from Womancare and its allies.

Responses and Change

Womancare staff, volunteers and allies were challenged to not only sustain services, but to ensure as safe an environment as possible for themselves and their patients. Specifically, organization members had to provide continued access to its services, offset financial losses, and counteract the various threats to reproductive rights. Yet rather than turning inward, as many clinics had done, Womancare engaged in aggressive marketing, service expansion, and advocacy efforts in order to deal with New Right actions.

Womancare staff and volunteers were trained in self-defense and safety measures, and private security guards were hired. All of these steps were financially costly; in 1986 (peak year for protesters) the Executive Director estimated that $150,000 went to security efforts alone. Womancare successfully used local noise ordinances to prevent protesters from "disturbing a hospital zone" and obtained court orders to keep picketers off clinic property. The emotional toll of New Right actions, especially those of the protesters, is more difficult to gauge. This Center report (1985) suggests, however, what clinic members went through:

> The demonstrators have viciously harassed clients, friends, staff and their children. We have added an escort service on Saturday mornings, including a shuttle service, utilizing community volunteers. Every Saturday we have had to hire an off-duty police officer. . . . We hired [an attorney] solely to assist us in fighting the anti-abortion attacks. Overall, the increase anti-abortion activity has added new stress to the entire staff and their families. . . . [With the arrival of Joe Scheidler] we started to feel what other clinics around the country were experiencing—paranoia (grounded in reality), frustration, shock and amazement at the fanaticism and perseverance of possessed, organized anti-abortion people.

The Center provided counseling and massages to staff and volunteers to help alleviate some of the anxiety and stress.

In order to generate greater revenue from clients, Womancare stream-lined its operations and focused its services to appeal to middle-class women. There was a distinct shift towards a more business emphasis:

> I think we need to recognize in our policymaking, fundraising and marketing that we are operating in a climate of conservatism, fis-cal and otherwise. . . . We cannot expect to continue doing what we are doing in the areas of fundraising and marketing and still con-tinue to grow. Everything I have heard about the future points to this larger picture. Te word is out. If you don't critically examine your organization as a business, your agency and your issue will not survive within the conservative agenda. (Executive Director, Report to the Board, 1987)

This shift, however, resulted in the loss of collectivist approaches to health care:

> In an effort to increase our business, we changed the structure of our Well Woman clinic. Women can now come in Mondays and Wednesdays, and are seen on an individual basis by a health worker and nurse practitioner. It seems as though more women are coming for services, and they are definitely here for a less amount of time. (Clinic report)

> We had to add on additional abortion clinics to generate money. We also had to appeal to a middle-class clientele that could pay. These women wanted privatized health care. We changed. The spiffier the clients, the spiffier we had to get. (Executive Director)

Corresponding to changes in program delivery, Womancare also devel-oped more hierarchical staffing arrangements and more bureaucratic approaches to communication and decision-making.

Womancare did maintain a commitment to its original self-help mis-sion, even if it was now longer operationalized in collectivist form:

> One of the most distinguishing features of Womancare is its status as the only non-profit clinic in the [metropolitan] area owned and operated by women–for women. More important, however, is the self-help philosophy that has guided the clinic since it began meet-ing the health care needs of women. Simply put: that sharing health care skills and information is the key to giving women more

control over their gynecological health and reproductive choices. (current brochure)

Perhaps even more important, the organization was able to eventually expand its range of program. After a brief period of service contraction, the 1990s saw considerable growth in Womancare offerings. Currently, the center provides abortions and abortion counseling, gynecological exams, pregnancy testing, infertility referrals, prenatal referrals, STD testing and treatment, breast health, birth control and emergency contraception options, breast health, donor insemination services and support groups, and HIV/AIDs testing and counseling (brochure). Indicators of a much stronger commitment to diversity include staff available to translate in Spanish, French, Hindi, Russian, Arabic, Urdu, Punjabi and Malay; special health programs designed for lesbian and bisexual, immigrant, younger, older, and disabled women; and the Homeless Women's Health Outreach Project. The Center also designed services specifically for survivors of sexual assault and incest.

One noticeable change was Womancare's outreach to other women's rights groups in the area. With their assistance, a clinic escort and shuttle system was established, so that clinic patients could get into the building. Overtime, these coalitions expanded to address issues such as violence against women, lesbian and gay rights, homelessness, welfare rights, and immigration. Womancare also formed alliances on the state and local level with more mainstream health enterprises and political groups, actions that never would have been engaged in during its founding period. For example, the Center served as a coalition leader in passing a cutting edge law prohibiting discrimination by insurance companies in covering birth control.

In terms of political action, the New Right provided an "external jolt" to Womancare. Strong anti-right rhetoric spilled forth from speeches, newsletter articles, and public testimonies:

> There is a war going on—a war between a woman's right to choose and fetal rights, between women's right to self-determination and fetus' "right to life." This war takes many forms including Medicaid payment cutoffs, parental consent requirements, picketing, marches on Washington, and clinic violence. . . . The feeling of this [the clinic attacks] instill in people who experience these acts is similar to the threat people feel from cross burnings or the use of swastikas. . . . Our biggest challenge is to swing the momentum

away from the anti-abortion perspective, away from "the silent scream" of the fetus to the woman's pain of an unwanted pregnancy and her need for privacy in such a personal matter. We must not compromise on abortion. . . . We must speak up for each woman's right to control her body and decide her future. (Executive Director, Speech to the National Lawyer's Guild)

Galvanized by the New Right, Womancare developed comprehensive programs for legislative advocacy, leadership training with particular emphasis on developing teen and young adult leaders, and community service. By 2003, the organization offered "Voice for Choice Training I & II," and "Citizen Lobbyist Training;" speaker bureau topics included "History of Abortion Rights," "Culturally Sensitive Counseling," Politics of Women's Health," "Effective Coalition Building," "Lesbian Health Care Issues," "Safer Sex," and "Empowering Gynecological Exams." These developments, together with the health services and coalition strategies, indicate an expansion of center offerings, even if the more explicit radical philosophy and processes had diminished.

DISCUSSION

In many respects, the story of Womancare is the story of the feminist health movement. Since the 1970s, there has been increased professionalization and institutionalization; processes that constrain the original version of collectivist approaches to health care. Yet the vision of self-help and advocacy for women's health remained. Moreover, the center, like the movement, expanded the issues it addressed and populations it served. It now more fully responds to the diverse needs and situations of women and girls. In doing so, Womancare illustrates how social change can be central feature in the delivery of human services (Heller, Price, Reinharz, Riger, & Wandersman, 1989; Morgenbesser, 1981; Withorn, 1984). Womancare's ability to survive captures the resilience of the feminist health movement, which is important since many of the accomplishments of this movement are now so well integrated into mainstream medical practice that they are taken for granted.

Womancare's continued existence rested on its strategy of engaging new constituent groups in the face of the sustained environmental threats. In doing so, it avoided a common pitfall of organizations in crisis, which is retreating rather than asserting itself in its environment

(Dyck, 1996; Helfgot, 1981; Warren, 1984). The ability of this center to determine new ways of enacting its mission through diversification provides a template for innovative nonprofit development.

The experiences of Womancare staff, patients and allies were not unique; feminist health centers across the country contended with similar oppositional efforts. To appreciate how extensive these threats were (and are), it is important to fully grasp the broader political context. Even though direct attacks by the New Right against Womancare began to ebb by the 1990s, for other women's health clinics, and even for more traditional reproductive health centers, the 1990s and into the 2000s remain times of intimidation, harassment and violence. The more harrowing anti-clinic actions included bomb threats and explosions, vandalism, shootings (7 of them fatal) of clinic staff, and anthrax scares (Bader & Baird-Windle, 2001; Bennett-Haigney, 1999; Clarkson, 2002; Feldt, 2004; Flanders, 2001; Lonsway et al., 2003). Through use of the internet, anti-choice activists posted "wanted dead or alive" posters of abortion providers and defended the "justifiable homicide" of reproductive health providers. One anti-abortion website, The Christian Gallery, is "a graphic of red, dripping blood and marks the doctors as working, wounded or fatalities. . . . Information on the doctors includes photographs, addresses, their children's names and ages, and other personal data;" it lists over 200 providers of and advocates for reproductive health services and essays such as "Why I shot an abortionist" by convicted killer Paul Hill (Bennett-Haigney, 1999). Threats and acts of violence were widespread, and even if a clinic was not directly attacked, it operated in an environment in which that was always a possibility.

There were pattern fluctuations in clinic violence, however, with the early 1990s continuing the trends of the 1980s. Under the Clinton administration, clinic violence was curtailed and federal investigation of incidents increased. Recent data suggests that as of 2001, coinciding with the start of the Bush administration, clinic violence re-escalated and federal investigations declined; overall, clinics reported multiple intimidation tactics were frequently used with bomb threats, stalking, death threats and blockades being the most common (Lonsway et al., 2003).

The last 15 years also have witnessed an increase in federal and state legislation that limits abortion and other reproductive health services. Since 1995, 380 state laws have been passed that restrict reproductive rights and services. As of 2003, 33 states have parental consent or notification laws, 36 states maintain Medicaid bans on abortion, and 19 states have mandatory waiting periods of 18 to 24 hours during which women must receive state-mandated lectures on the risks of abortions.

For over a decade, Congress has barred military hospitals from offering abortions, even if the woman's life is in danger. It is generally believed that the next appointment to the U.S. Supreme Court will determine the fate of legalized abortion nationally (Bader & Baird-Windle, 2001; Feldt, 2004; National Organization for Women, 2004).

The combination of direct violence and legislation has had the effect of severely curtailing the availability of abortions. Only 13% of all U.S. counties have an abortion provider. One third of American cities have no reproductive health centers, and rural areas are even more limited. Less than half of all medical schools train students in first-trimester abortions (Bader & Baird-Windle, 2001; Feldt, 2004; Morgen, 2002; Ruzek, 1998). These events suggest a significant erosion of health care, especially for women and girls. Moreover, because proponents of reproductive choice must continuously fight oppositional measures, there are insufficient resources to promote or enact initiatives aimed at expanding health coverage to more vulnerable groups of women (National Organization for Women, 2004).

The stories of Womancare, specifically, and the feminist health movement, in general, hold larger implications for health policy and practice. Factors such as health consumer rights groups, the training and availability of competent medical personnel, technological advances, managed care, and the debates concerning universal coverage all impinge upon the implementation of policy initiatives (Kronenfeld, 2000; Magner, 1996; Segal & Brzuzy, 1998). What Womancare so strikingly illustrates is how oppositional forces (New Right) directly and indirectly altered the availability of legal and legitimate health options. Understanding what health organizations such as Womancare endure sheds light on the highly politicized nature of health care in this country.

The legal right to abortion, and any other health service, is hollow if access is not protected. Yet efforts to close down this center, and similar clinics, are not solely about the issue of abortion, even though its legalization and availability are at the heart of the feminist health movement. As Feldt asserts, "the right to have full access to family planning information, facilities, and products, the right to have children or not, . . . and the right to medically accurate information" are endangered (2004, p. 9). The Womancare Health Center, and the feminist health movement as a whole, serves as a cautionary tale about the precarious provision of health care in this country.

CONCLUSION

To contend with a challenging environment, the Womancare Health Center developed strategies for sustaining its health care goals. Specifically, Center members responded to oppositional efforts by expanding and diversifying its health services, educational programs, and outreach activities. In doing so, the Womancare Health Center offers a template for sustaining the social policy goals of open access to women's health care services in the face of often hostile and well-mobilized political and social forces.

NOTE

1. To insure confidentiality and anonymity, "Womancare" is a pseudonym and some details associated with the organization and its members have been altered. Data for this case study, gathered and analyzed by the author, are from interviews with center members, documents, and observations.

REFERENCES

Bader, E., & Baird-Windle, P. (2001). *Targets of hatred: Anti-abortion terrorism.* New York: Macmillan.

Baird, K. (1998). *Gender justice and the health care system.* New York: Garland.

Bennett-Haigney, L. (1999). *Doctor murdered as anti-abortion violence and terrorism continue.* Retrieved May 22, 2005, from www.now.org/nnt/winter-99/aborvio.html

Boston Women's Health Book Collective. (2005). *Our bodies, ourselves: A new edition for a new era* (35th anniversary ed.). New York: Touchstone.

Clarkson, F. (2002). *Anti-abortion terrorism threatens all Americans.* Retrieved May 22, 2005, from www.commondreams.org

Dailard, C. (2001). Challenges facing family planning clinics and Title X. *The Guttmacher Report on Public Policy, 4*(2), 1-26.

Dixon-Miller, R. (1993). *Population policy and women's rights: Transforming reproductive choice.* Westport, CT: Praeger.

Dyck, B. (1996). The role of crises and opportunities in organizational change: A look at a nonprofit religious college. *Nonprofit and Voluntary Sector Quarterly, 25*(3), 321-446.

Ehrenreich, B., & English, D. (1979). *For her own good.* Garden City: Anchor Books.

Feldt, G. (2004). *The war on choice: The right-wing attack on women's rights and how to fight back.* New York: Bantam.

Feminist Women's Health Center. (2000). *Firebombs and violence.* Retrieved May 22, 2005, 2005, from www.fwhc.org/firebombs.htm

Flanders, L. (2001). *Unsung heroes.* Retrieved May 22, 2005, from www.workingforchange. com

Geary, M. A. (1995). An analysis of the women's health movement and its impact on the delivery of health care within the United States. *The Nurse Practitioner, 20*(11).

Gelb, J., & Palley, M. L. (1996). *Women and public policies.* Charlottesville, VA: The University of Virginia Press.

Gillespie, E., Gingrich, N., Schellhas, B., & Armey, R. (Eds.). (1994). *Contract with America.* New York: Three Rivers Press.

Helfgot, J. (1981). *Professional reforming.* Lexington, MA: Lexington Books.

Heller, K., Price, R., Reinharz, S., Riger, S., & Wandersman, A. (1989). *Psychology and community change* (2nd ed.). Boston: Wadsworth Publishing.

Hyde, C. (1992). The ideational system of social movement agencies: An examination of feminist health centers. In Y. Hasenfeld (Ed.), *Human services as complex organizations* (pp. 121-144). Newbury Park, CA: Sage Publications.

Hyde, C. (1995). Feminist social movement organizations survive the new right. In M. M. Ferree & P. Y. Martin (Eds.), *Feminist organizations: Harvest of the new women's movement* (pp. 306-322). Philadelphia, PA: Temple University Press.

Kolk, A. (1996). Gender perspectives and quality of care: Towards appropriate and adequate health care for women. *Social Science and Medicine, 43*(5), 708-725.

Kraynak, M. A. (1994). The women's health movement: Political, social and medical issues. *American Pharmacy, NS34*(12), 30-35.

Kronenfeld, J. (2000). Social policy and health care. In J. Midgely, M. Tracey, & M. Livermore (Eds.), *The handbook of social policy* (pp. 221-236). Thousand Oaks, CA: Sage Publications.

Lonsway, K., Jackman, J., Koenig, E., Leader, J., & Campos, P. (2003). *2002 National Clinic Violence Survey Report.* Washington, DC: Feminist Majority Foundation.

Lundy, M., & Mason, S. (1994). Women's health care centers: Multiple definitions. *Social Work in Health Care, 19*(3/4), 109-122.

Magner, G. (1996). Health care and rationing. In P. Raffoul & C. McNeece (Eds.), *Future issues for social work practice* (pp. 39-48). Boston: Allyn & Bacon.

Morgen, S. (1990). Contradictions in feminist practice: Individualism and collectivism in a feminist health center. *Comparative Social Research, Supplement, 1*, 9-59.

Morgen, S. (2002). *Into our own hands: The women's health movement in the United States, 1969-1990.* New Brunswick, NJ: Rutgers University Press.

Morgenbesser, M. (1981). The evolution of three alternative social service agencies. *Catalyst, 11*, 71-83.

National Organization for Women. (2004). *Reproductive rights steadily eroded in the states.* Retrieved May 22, 2005, from www.now.org/issues/abortion/031704states.html

Nichols, F. H. (2000). History of the women's health movement in the 20th century. *Journal of Obstetric, Gynecological and Neonatal Nursing, 29*(1), 56-64.

Palley, M. L., & Palley, H. (2000). Rethinking a women's health care agenda. *Women & Politics, 21*(3), 75-99.

Phillips, B. (1996). *Salvi guilty but clinics still under fire.* Retrieved May 22, 2005, from www.now.org/nnt/05-96/salvi.html

Ratcliff, K. (2002). *Women and health: Power, technology, inequality and conflict in a gendered world.* Boston: Allyn & Bacon.

Reproductive Rights National Network. (1978, Summer). Bill of reproductive rights *Reproductive Rights News,* p. 2.

Rosser, S. (2002). An overview of women's health in the U.S. since the mid-1960s. *History and Technology, 18*(4), 355-369.

Ruzek, S. B. (1978). *The women's health movement: Feminist alternatives to medical control.* New York: Praeger Publishers.

Ruzek, S. B. (1998). *The women's health movement from the 1960s to the present, and beyond.* Retrieved April 27, 2005, from www.4woman.gov/owh/pub/history/healthmvmt.htm

Ruzek, S. B. (2004). How might the women's health movement shape national agendas on women and aging? *Women's Health Issues, 14,* 112-114.

Scheidler, J. (1985). *Closed: 99 ways to stop abortion.* Wheaton, IL: Crossway Books.

Segal, E., & Brzuzy, S. (1998). *Social welfare policy, programs, and practice.* Itasca, IL: F.E. Peacock Publishers.

Sherwin, S. (Ed.). (1998). *The politics of women's health: Exploring agency and autonomy.* Philadelphia: Temple University Press.

Warren, D. (1984). Managing in crisis: Nine principles for successful transition. In J. Kimberly & R. Quinn (Eds.), *New futures: The challenge of managing corporate transitions* (pp. 85-106). Homewood, IL: Dow Jones-Irwin.

Weinstein, M., & Clark, L. (1998). *NOW mobilizes in wake of deadly clinic bombing.* Retrieved May 22, 2005, from www.now.org/nnt/03-98/brmnghm.html

Weisman, C. (1998). *Women's health care: Activist tradition and institutional change.* Baltimore: The Johns Hopkins University Press.

Weisman, C., Curbow, B., & Khoury, A. (1995). The national survey of women's health centers: Current models of women-centered care. *Women's Health Issues, 5*(3), 103-117.

Withorn, A. (1984). *Serving the people: Social services and social change.* New York: Columbia University Press.

Zimmerman, M., & Hill, S. (2000). Reforming gendered health care: An assessment of change. *International Journal of Health Services, 30*(4), 771-795.

The Voice of Advocates in Health Care Policymaking for the Poor

Colleen M. Grogan

Michael K. Gusmano

INTRODUCTION

When a state legislature creates an intentionally inclusive advisory committee to discuss the design and implementation of a new health care program for poor families, what topics are discussed? Do they actively engage in conversation around the agreed upon goals for the new reform? In Connecticut, the legislature and the participants of the Council and its sub-committees agreed that the goals of Medicaid managed care (MMC) were threefold: (1) to reduce the costs of the program; (2) to improve the quality of health care recipients receive; and, (3) to increase access to mainstream health care services. While there was substantial public discussion about the first two goals, there was very little talk about the third goal. Participants in the various public forums that we observed over an eighteen-month period had difficultly discussing whether and how MMC would give poor families access to mainstream health care services. The lack of discussion was not because participants thought the issue was unimportant or even less important than the other two goals. Ironically, in our private interviews participants mentioned access to mainstream health care most often as the most important challenge of MMC.

The purpose of this chapter is to document this central puzzle that emerges from our findings: what the majority of participants said they cared most about privately, they were least able to discuss publicly. We begin by providing a brief background about the emergence of Medicaid managed care in Connecticut and the participatory process, and discuss our methods to study this process. We then turn to our findings and begin by showing the fluidity of discussion around the first two goals–costs and quality–and contrast that with the vividly strained and truncated discussion around the goal of equal access to health care services. We juxtapose our findings of the public discussion with the findings from our private interviews with participants to illustrate our puzzle of private concern and public silence. Next we present possible reasons for the emergence of this puzzle, and conclude by considering what these findings imply about the development of social policy in health care.

HOPE IN MEDICAID MANAGED CARE: 1990s

In the early 1990s, policymakers readily characterized state Medicaid programs as administrative failures. To be sure, most policymakers acknowledged that Medicaid played a crucial role in providing health coverage for millions of Americans. Yet there was broad agreement–among Republican and Democratic officials alike–that Medicaid suffered from serious operational flaws. Medicaid still failed to cover many needy persons, and the health care it offered was too often of low quality and provided inefficiently. Numerous studies documented that Medicaid recipients were much *less* likely than Americans with private health insurance to have a relationship with a primary care doctor or to receive needed preventive care, and much *more* likely to receive their care in hospital emergency room settings or public clinics with long waiting lines (Davidson & Somers, 1988; CRS, 1993). Despite the targeted efforts to increase pre-natal care and well childcare coverage in the 1980s, a large proportion of Medicaid women still received no, or only minimal, pre-natal care services (Colburn, 1991). Many children enrolled in Medicaid were failing to receive needed immunizations (Slovut, 1991). Layered atop these concerns about health care access and quality were concerns about Medicaid costs. While the annual growth rate of Medicaid spending declined immediately following the retrenchment period in the early 1980s, Medicaid costs rose steadily thereafter. As the program expansions for children and pregnant women and other legislative changes for the elderly and disabled adopted in the 1980s and early 1990s were phased-in along with fee increases, Medicaid expenditures shot up (Coughlin, Ku, & Holahan, 1994: 48-51; Rowland, Feder, & Salganicoff, 1993).

Yet if Medicaid spending was growing rapidly in the 1990s, so too were the ranks of the uninsured.[1] Many policymakers argued that it was inequitable to provide Medicaid coverage to the non-working poor at a time when two-thirds of uninsured Americans came from families with at least one working parent (Beamer, 1999). When Medicaid was originally created, the assumption was that aid should be offered to those who could not afford health insurance because of their lack of employment (U.S. Senate, 1967: 1547). By the 1990s, however, it was widely acknowledged that being employed does not guarantee affordable health insurance coverage (Blendon, Young & DesRoches, 1999). The inability of the working poor to obtain affordable health insurance further promoted the view that Medicaid should be a program distinct from welfare.

States were encouraged by incentives offered through federal Medicaid waivers to "solve" these problems by implementing Medicaid Managed Care (MMC). In 1993, President Clinton ordered the federal government to make it easier for state to use Medicaid funds to introduce new health care programs for low-income families. The federal Health Care

Financing Administration streamlined its waiver application process so that more states could implement Medicaid managed care reforms (Friedman, 1993). National policymakers promoted the managed care approach almost as a "magic bullet" solution: it promised simultaneously to reduce costs, improve access, raise the quality of delivered services, and even expand coverage to the uninsured (Grogan, 1997; Hurley & Somers, 2003).

Given the intense pressures they faced to improve Medicaid services, rein in program costs and expand access to the uninsured, state Medicaid policymakers were eager to experiment with this new administrative approach. By January 1995 each of the fifty states (except Alaska) had implemented a Medicaid managed care program. Nationally, total enrollment in Medicaid managed care nearly doubled in 1994 and increased 51 percent again in 1995 (Horvath & Kaye, 1995; Grogan, 1997). States under Democratic legislative control were just as eager to implemented managed care reforms as were states under Republican legislative control. Ideological and other political factors were swamped by the appeal of reduced costs, increased access and improved quality of care.

Under Medicaid managed care, states contract with Managed Care Organizations (MCOs) at 95 percent of the current cost to run their Medicaid programs. Each state pays MCOs a pre-set monthly amount for each member in the plan whether or not the member actually utilizes any medical care services during the month. The theory is that MCOs make money by emphasizing preventive care and reducing unnecessary utilization of expensive medical services, such as preventable emergency room use. Efficient MCOs, for example, may be able to provide services at only 85 percent of the cost baseline, allowing them to retain the 10 percent difference.[2]

There was also hope that Medicaid managed care would achieve mainstream access (Iglehart, 1999). In particular, by contracting with Managed Care Organizations (MCOs) policymakers hope that MCOs will use their market-based leverage (and other strategies such as increasing fees) to convince commercial providers to participate in the Medicaid program (Holahan et al., 1998). Findings from Holahan et al.'s (1998) analysis of Medicaid managed care programs in 13 states illustrate this point:

> They (policymakers) doubt that higher rates will increase the number of Medicaid providers. The state officials with whom we spoke see a greater likelihood of improved access if managed care plans

are required to attract and retain an adequate number of providers (p. 44-45).

Similarly, Oliver (1998) concludes from his study of Medicaid managed care in Maryland that many reformers view the use of managed care contracting as an opportunity to open up access to mainstream providers and services.

Medicaid advocates also appear to frequently support Medicaid managed care specifically because they view such reforms as an opportunity to overcome the stigma associated with the traditional Medicaid program. For example, the director of a Phoenix-based philanthropy touts Arizona's Medicaid managed care program because "many Medicaid patients have access to mainstream private physicians whom they did not previously have access to. They don't feel like charity patient's anymore" (Iglehart, 1995). And, consumer advocate, Geraldine Dalleck, from Families USA Foundation, writes "Medicaid managed care may offer the last, best opportunity to provide integrated health care for the nation's poor (Dalleck, 1996).

CONNECTICUT'S HOPE IN MMC: 1993-1995

A number of factors contributed to Connecticut's interest in Medicaid managed care. Perhaps most significant were the state's fiscal crisis in the early 1990s and the rapid growth of its Medicaid program between 1985 and 1994. Like many other states, particularly those in the northeast and California, Connecticut continued to feel the effects of the 1990-1991 national recession for a few years after it ended in March 1991 (Gold, 1996). And, as in many of these other states, Connecticut's economic slowdown and state budget crisis were exacerbated by the growth of the state's Medicaid program. Between 1985 and 1994, total state Medicaid expenditures jumped from $5 million to roughly $1.6 billion (Connecticut General Assembly, 1994: 21). The number of persons eligible for Medicaid increased by 31 percent between 1991 and 1994. In contrast to the general fund budget, which increased by 20 percent, the state's Medicaid budget increased by 35 percent between 1991 and 1994 (Connecticut General Assembly, 1994: 22). Because the Medicaid program represented roughly one quarter of Connecticut's General Fund, the growth in Medicaid costs had a dramatic effect on the budget. This generated a considerable amount of interest in containing Medicaid costs.

However, Connecticut's Medicaid officials were also interested in expanding access to care for the program's recipients, and they thought that managed care would help them achieve this goal. Similar to the long-standing goals throughout Medicaid's history, they were concerned that recipients were not receiving needed services of sufficient quality. During our interviews, officials articulated two reasons why they believed that private Managed Care Organizations (MCOs) could do a better job of expanding access to services for the Medicaid population. First, they thought that MCOs would have more resources for outreach. State Medicaid officials claimed that under the fee-for-service program, the Governor and General Assembly had been unwilling to appropriate enough funds to the department for effective outreach to the Medicaid population.

Second, the Connecticut Medicaid officials believed that MCOs would be more effective in encouraging physicians to participate in the Medicaid program. For years state officials had been frustrated by the low participation rates of physicians, particularly pediatricians and obstetricians. They believed that MCOs were in a better position to expand physician participation because they would have more leverage over providers. MCOs could, in theory, make participation in their private insurance networks contingent upon the willingness of physicians to accept the plan's Medicaid patients.

Finally, officials wanted to adopt managed care because of the perception that Connecticut was lagging behind other "innovative" states. By 1994, the vast majority of states had implemented some form of Medicaid managed care. In December 1994, even after the General Assembly had passed a Medicaid managed care bill, the state's main newspaper, *The Hartford Courant*, chided the state for failing to follow this trend. "This state is wasting money by using an expensive system that others have abandoned. This trend toward a 'managed-care' health care network has taken hold in most places except at Connecticut's Medicaid offices . . . Only two other states have not adopted managed care for Medicaid patients" (Williams, 1994).

Officials in DSS were sensitive to these criticisms and anxious to move forward. As one member of the Department put it, "we were aware that we had lagged behind what had been done in some other states. So we were thinking about what could we do that would kind of boost us forward." In 1992, DSS commissioned a study of the Medicaid managed care (MMC) programs of other states with the intent of learning from their experiences. Bolstered by other states' favorable experiences, the General Assembly created a managed care division in the

Department of Social Services (DSS). By 1993, the Medicaid Director had created a Medicaid managed care advisory committee comprised primarily of representatives from the managed care industry. According to DSS officials, the primary purpose of the advisory committee was to provide the department with feedback about the design of the new program, and, in so doing, to generate interest and commitment among HMOs to participate in the program.

The makeup of this advisory committee was purposely limited. It included representatives from HMOs and Community Health Centers (CHCs),[3] and only one Medicaid advocate.[4] The Department did not want to involve a broader set of actors until they had developed the basic design of the program. DSS officials believed that opposition to managed care from Medicaid advocates would have poisoned the atmosphere and discouraged plans from participating in the Medicaid program. Clearly, by DSS's own admission, this advisory committee did not represent an open or inclusive process.

Of course, interested groups that were excluded criticized this closed process. Critics asserted that the process was both unfair and insufficient because it left out "core constituencies" (Grogan & Gusmano, 2005). Toward the end of 1993, the advisory committee dissolved in the face of opposition from Medicaid advocates and others who argued that the decision making process was too industry focused.

In response, DSS began a "diplomacy campaign." In early 1994, DSS held nearly 30 meetings throughout the state with provider groups and advocates. In May 1994, DSS held a conference on Medicaid managed care attended by over more than 240 individuals, and met with more than 300 different organizations including other state agencies, provider groups, managed care plans and advocacy organizations to answer questions about the reform proposal.[5] During these meetings, DSS articulated a clear set of objectives for the Medicaid managed care initiative, which were very consistent with long held goals for Medicaid across the states and over time–equal access, improved quality and cost control. According to DSS, the initiative was designed to improve health, expand access to care, promote continuity of care and reduce long-term Medicaid costs. DSS placed great emphasis on the capacity of managed care to promote growth of delivery networks. Among the criteria DSS claimed it would use to evaluate managed care plans were their ability to include historical Medicaid providers and their ability to bring *"new points of access to Medicaid eligibles"* (DSS PowerPoint presentation, Legislative Office Building, Hartford, CT, August 23, 1994; *emphasis* added by authors).

Because the purpose of the diplomacy campaign was to persuade, and there was no effort to involve groups in a discussion about policy design, Medicaid advocates and Medicaid providers were frustrated and dissatisfied with the decision making process and made their views known to key elected officials in the state legislature. In response to these concerns, the legislature gave DSS authority to submit a waiver to the federal government to implement a Medicaid Managed Care (MMC) program, but prohibited the implementation of the program for one year, so that a newly created twenty-six member Medicaid Managed Care Council could deliberate on the design of the program as well as the implementation.[6] Specifically, DSS was required to provide the Council with monthly reports on its plans for implementation of Medicaid managed care. In turn, the MMC Council would discuss the proposals and advise the DSS.

The MMC Council met monthly. Council members included Medicaid advocates, provider representatives, health plan executives, Medicaid consumers, state legislators, and state agency representatives. The Council created four subcommittees focusing on different issue areas: Access, Quality Assurance, Public Health, and Behavioral (Mental/Substance Abuse) Health. These four subcommittees also held monthly meetings. In addition to the MMC Council, the General Assembly created the Connecticut Children's Health Project (CCHP) to monitor the impact of MMC on Medicaid children. The CCHP created the Children's Health Council and it also held monthly meetings.

Thus, with the Children's Health Council, the MMC Council and its four subcommittees there were sixty-four public meetings, in just one year, devoted specifically to discussing Medicaid managed care reform. Their main collective function was to act as deliberative bodies—discussing whether the design and implementation of Medicaid managed care lived up to the agreed upon goals of improving quality, expanding access to care, and cost control.

FINDINGS

Public Talk About Health Care Reform for the Poor

Access to Mainstream Physicians

Starting in August of 1995, AFDC-Medicaid recipients living in Connecticut's two largest counties[7] were given the option to enroll in a

Medicaid managed care plan. Recipients' response to the new program was extraordinary: by the end of the month, nearly ten thousand Medicaid recipients had enrolled in eleven different Medicaid MCOs. The number of voluntary enrollments was far greater than anyone–including the agency responsible for administering the program (the Department of Social Services–DSS), Medicaid advocates, and the MCOs–anticipated.

Not surprisingly, especially given this level of unanticipated demand, a number of enrollment difficulties arose during the first few months of the program. Medicaid Managed Care (MMC) Council members–many of whom worked on some aspect of the program–shared anecdotes about the poor quality of information available to Medicaid recipients, and worried about the extent to which recipients were making informed choices. Early in the implementation stage, in a January 1996 meeting, many Council members raised concerns that Medicaid recipients were making uninformed choices. Medicaid advocates were specifically worried that Medicaid recipients were choosing commercial plans under the belief they were getting a commercial product (i.e., access to more "mainstream" private providers) when, in fact, they were getting a separate Medicaid-MCO plan. For example, Blue Cross Blue Shield of Connecticut created a Medicaid plan called "Bluecare" that has a list of providers, which is different from the list of providers a private paying subscriber would get. The commercial insurers' Medicaid plans had many "traditional" Medicaid providers (primarily those practicing in public clinics), as well as "new" private physicians on their Medicaid panels, but the extent to which private providers actually participated was unknown. While there were many new private physicians listed as participating in MMC, there was no information on the *extent* of provider participation in the program. For example, a physician could be listed as available on an MCO's brochure, but only see one or two Medicaid patients in any given year. Moreover, there was some concern about the validity of the MCO lists because there were reports of some physicians on the lists that had no idea they were listed and had no intention of seeing a Medicaid patient. This happened because some MCOs had very lenient physician participation rules. For example, one MCO simply sent all its private physicians a letter stating that the plan would add the physician to its Medicaid list of participating providers unless the plan heard back from the physician stating that s/he did not want to be listed–a type of "regrets only" participation rule. This approach combined with the lack of data about how and whether physicians were actually participating in MMC created two divergent views about the access goal: some look at the lists and said that MMC created access to mainstream providers, others doubted the accuracy of the lists and thought MCOs were simply creating a false image.

In the January meeting, several explicit concerns about equitable treatment were raised. For example, one state Senator said he was aware of differences between the commercial networks and Medicaid networks, thought it unfair to Medicaid recipients, and "believed the plans should do a better job encouraging commercial providers to join the Medicaid networks (#75)."[8] Another state legislator said, "Many who have voluntarily chosen a plan think they selected the BCBS commercial plan, but they have not. When they do find out there is a big difference, they are having problems (#16)." Representatives of the poor provided there own anecdotes, which suggested the state was unfairly misleading recipients into thinking they were getting more from MCOs than they were actually given. For example, a Medicaid advocate said she had visited housing projects and talked with clients "who have chosen BCBS, but did not understand what they were getting (#71)."

While many members were concerned about equitable treatment given the existence of separate Medicaid networks, the conversation abruptly ended when a representative from BCBS said "there are more providers in our Medicaid network (under this new managed care reform) than had served the population under Medicaid's previous FFS program (#54)." In our private interviews, advocates for the poor often raised the issue of provider participation in the Medicaid managed care plans as a central issue of concern. They worried that, despite the rhetoric, a two-tiered system of care that long existed under Medicaid was being replicated under this new reform. Yet, once the incremental claim–that this reform program is an improvement over the previous status quo–was launched in the public forum, discussion about how well the program was achieving this goal ended. Indeed, this particular issue was never raised again during the remaining sixteen months of the public meetings that we observed.

Access to Mainstream Dentists

Discussion about improving access to health care services under MMC continued in the Access Sub-committee–as one would hope and expect given its title. While members of the subcommittee had concerns about access to medical care more generally, they focused their attention on access to dental services. Dental care was a serious problem in the MMC program. Very few private, mainstream dentists participated in the program. This was the case prior to the managed care reform, but access actually worsened after the implementation of managed care because dentists in Connecticut were particularly hostile to working and contracting with MCOs. Thus, not only were dentists reluctant to take Medicaid patients, they did not want to deal with MCOs either. The access subcommittee strategized about ways to improve dental access with a very immediate goal of having at least as many dentists in the program as that which participated prior to the MMC reform.

To increase dental participation in the program, they primarily focused their efforts on an initiative to standardize administrative practices among MCOs. Because each of the eleven MCOs in the program required a different administrative process for dentists to contract with their MCO, dentists often commented that the administrative process associated with the MMC reform was overly burdensome. Thus, subcommittee participants worked extremely hard with both dentists and MCOs in an effort to create a common administrative process across plans so that the administrative burden would not deter dentists, who might ordinarily participate in the Medicaid program.

Of course, the main purpose of managed care is to "manage" patient care, and MCOs use their administrative forms as a way to keep track of patient utilization and provider practices. Thus, the way providers report information to MCOs is extremely important to the MCO and often considered proprietary information. As a result, what might at first blush appear to be a relatively easy policy solution to implement turned out to be quite difficult because MCOs participating in Connecticut's program were very resistant to creating a common administrative form. Hence, what might be perceived as a trivial achievement from an outside perspective was viewed by participants in the deliberative process as an important feat. As a provider representative (not a dentist), announced publicly to the MMC Council: "the access problem for dental services has been grappled with in the Access subcommittee . . . The subcommittee is trying to develop one claim form for all dental services and one credentialing form for all plans and providers. *It has not been easy*."

After the Access subcommittee's success in securing a common administrative form for dentists, the behavioral health subcommittee began also working on a common administrative form to increase participation among mental health providers in the program. Indeed, advocates with concerns about lack of providers funneled their interests into this very specific solution. If they could make it easier for providers to participate in Connecticut's MMC program, thereby increasing access for Medicaid recipients, this was viewed as a worthwhile endeavor.

Besides creating a common administrative form, Access subcommittee participants also focused on how to increase the ability of *public-funded* clinics to provide needed dental care. As mentioned in chapter two, the lack of providers willing to participate in state Medicaid programs has been a problem almost since the program began in 1965. Low reimbursement rates, negative provider perceptions of Medicaid recipients, and administrative burden, have long been identified as reasons why physicians do not participate in state Medicaid programs. In response to the lack of participation, the federal government has long supported the development of publicly funded clinics to take care of the uninsured, as well as Medicaid patients. Publicly funded Community Health Centers (CHCs) are a prominent source of primary care for the uninsured in America. However, due to the lack of physicians will to participate in state Medicaid programs, CHCs have also been an important source of care for Medicaid enrollees. Indeed, about half of the CHC clients in Connecticut were Medicaid eligible. Another source of care for children that has developed over the last twenty to thirty years are School-based Health Centers (SBHCs). A central idea behind both CHCs and SBHCs is that they will be able to provide preventive care more effectively by bringing the care to where the people are–in underserved communities, and in their schools. SBHCs rely heavily on nurse practitioners to provide preventive health care and dental hygienists to provide preventive dental care.

Thus, looking toward expanding the capacity of public clinics to "solve" the lack of dental participation in Connecticut's Medicaid program is not a new idea, and some argued counterproductive to the access goals specified under MMC. In particular, because many proponents of MMC argued that this reform provides an opportunity for Medicaid recipients to access "mainstream" providers and services (Holahan, 1998; Dalleck, 1996; Oliver, 1996), this fallback to the public clinic approach was viewed by many as problematic.

There are many reasons why MMC is viewed as having the potential to improve provider participation in Medicaid. One main reason is based on states holding MCOs accountable. Indeed, MCO accountability was the main lever that people looked to in Connecticut. The state imposed specific provider-to-patient ratios. When MCOs did not meet the ratio requirement–that is, the MCO had too few physicians, for example, compared to Medicaid enrollees–within a specific county, that state would withhold any further enrollment in the plan (within that county) until the MCO is able to increase the number of physicians will to participate in that county. These ratios applied to both primary care physicians and dentists.

On the dental side, many plans–especially in certain counties–were having difficulty enrolling enough dentists to meet the ratio require- ment. As a result, the state withheld additional enrollments into those MCOs in counties where the MCO was not meeting the ratio require- ment. For the ratio requirement, the only providers that counted were dentists. This raised some concerns because although some plans con- tracted with SBHCs that used dental hygienists, DSS did not count den- tal hygienists as "providers" in their calculation of the dental ratio requirement.

DSS argued–and many advocates and others agreed–that although dental hygienists in SBHCs provided good and needed services, it was also important that Medicaid enrollees have access to dentists–"just like the general population"–several participants said aloud. These partici- pants wanted to keep the ratio requirement for dentists to force plans to increase the number of participating dentists. Other participants openly disagreed with this perspective in the public forum. They acknowledge that having more dentists in the system would be ideal, but were pessi- mistic that the ratio requirement would make any difference given the long-standing problems of getting dentists to participate in Medicaid. They argued, pragmatically, that by including dental hygienists in SBHCs in the ratio requirement, plans would see the potential of SBHCs for ex- panding access, and SBHCs with dental clinics would be able to expand capacity, thus increasing access to dental services for Medicaid eligible children. For example, in the MMC Council, a provider representative said:

> What about counting mid-level providers such as dental hygien- ists? If employed in a public health setting, could they be counted as providers by DSS in the 1:486 ratio? We could also promote SBHCs (MMC Council Meeting; June, 1996).

In direct contrast from this view, those who favored only counting dentists in the ratio requirement believed that changing the ratio to in- clude dental hygienists would just be a counting gimmick. Since the plans were already required to contract with SBHCs (through another provision in their contract with DSS), it would not 'truly' expand access for Medicaid children. And, in the meantime, they reasoned, it would let the health plans "off the hook."

I don't see how this helps improve access. It's just a counting issue. SBHC and CHCs already at capacity so if anything it helps the plans that have had trouble getting dentists (Medicaid Advocate; MMC Council Meeting; June, 1996)

After discussing the issue in the Council's June meeting, a member of the Medicaid Managed Care Council presented a resolution in July of 1996 from the Access subcommittee that called upon the Department of Social Services to promote the use of School Based Health Centers (SBHC)–a publicly funded program staffed largely by dental hygienists. Obviously, the intent was to increase the use of dental services for Medicaid children. After presenting the resolution, the following discussion ensued.

State Bureaucrat (#90): "I wonder about a professionalized dental care system which encourages particular types of care in certain venues. I wonder whether or not this might create a two-tiered system. Whether adoption of this type of resolution will then let dentists in private offices off the hook."

State Representative (#61): "Having worked in a SBHC, I can say unequivocally, that it is not a two-tiered system. It happens to be comparable. Full services are provided, and when needed they are referred on to a private dentist. At no time do I feel that their services are compromised. In fact, what would happen if this method was not offered is they would get no services at all."

State Bureaucrat (#90): "Again if you look at the current arrangement, there is already a contractual requirement with the managed care plans to contract with the SBHCs. I just raise the issue of whether it is right to go further with this emphasis. I think SBHCs do a good job; it is just a question of particular emphasis.

State Representative (#61): "But, private dentists don't participate. We know what the problems are, and this is a strategy to solve the problem. It is an adjunct to that."

MCO Representative (#42): "I understand that SBHCs work, but this takes pressure off private providers and managed care plans."

Medicaid Advocate (#17): "As I said in the beginning [when she presented the resolution], this was seen as part of an overall strategy recognizing that [getting dentists to participate] is incredibly problematic. And, in fact, I think we recognized this in the first place when we discussed carving out dental services [separating dental services from the MMC program]. In a sense, by including it [dental services in the capitation rate] we hoped, in a way, that we could make the managed care plans accountable for providing dental services. But, they have the same problem with getting providers to participate that people in the Medicaid program had before."

State Senator (#58): "One of the things that comes to mind for me is that there are no easy answers. With Medicaid, people are not getting the health care that they need, they haven't ever, and they still aren't." [Medicaid Managed Care Council Meeting, July 19, 1996]

Given the history of Medicaid, and health care services to the poor more generally, it is not surprising that participants–as the State Senator suggested–were skeptical and pessimistic that any real change in mainstreaming would occur. Indeed, participants–even those who disagreed with the resolution in principle–decided to focus strategically on what they thought they could achieve–increase the capacity of public clinics for Medicaid recipients. All but one member of the Council voted in favor of adopting the resolution. Then, after the vote, their attention was diverted to other matters. The discussion about a two-tiered system, and how to hold plans accountable for provider participation to create a one-tiered system–all the important topics around the goal of improving access to mainstream services–was again dropped from further public discussion.

Health Plan Participation in MMC

By February of 1996, when program participation was mandatory statewide, the Department of Social Services (DSS) had signed contracts with eleven MCOs. Six of these were commercial "brand-name" insurance plans that created separate Medicaid programs when submitting their bids to the state. The remaining five MCOs were called Medicaid-only plans because traditional Medicaid providers created them for the sole purpose of providing services to Medicaid recipients (i.e., these plans had no commercial subscribers). Concern about the effect of MMC reform on these traditional Medicaid providers, also called safety-net providers, received a good deal of public attention.

As mentioned, due to the lack of physicians willing to participate in Connecticut's Medicaid program, the state has long relied on Community Health Centers (CHCs) as a key source of health care for Medicaid recipients. Besides Medicaid enrollees, CHCs are also an important source of care for persons without health insurance (CITE). Indeed,

CHCs structure the health care they provide around the special needs of their clientele (CITE). In efforts to reduce not just the financial barriers to accessing health care for the poor, but also the non-financial barriers, CHCs provide the following types of "enabling" services: translation services for non-English speakers, transportation to the facility so appointments are kept, walk-in appointments are allowed, and referral services to other social services agencies.

The federal government recognized the importance of these additional "enabling" services provided by CHCs by increasing their Medicaid reimbursement rate in 1989 (to what is called "cost-based reimbursement"). Many CHCs claimed that they relied on Medicaid cost-based reimbursement to help subsidize the care they provided to the uninsured. Indeed, in the CHCs in Connecticut, Medicaid made up about half of the patient population (Grogan & Gusmano, 1999).

When Connecticut switched to MMC, many–including CHCs themselves–feared CHCs would have financial difficulties for two reasons. First, there is no requirement under MMC that health plans must pay CHCs the higher cost-based reimbursement. (Indeed, as feared, most plans paid the lower reimbursement that other providers received.) Second, some worried that CHCs may lose some of their Medicaid client base and thus have an even larger proportion of self-pay, uninsured patients. With these two points in mind, there was a debate among the CHCs as to whether they should contract with participating MCOs or create their own MCO.

In the end, they decided to create their own MCO for three reasons. First, CHCs did not want to be beholden to commercial insurers and their notion of "appropriate utilization." Second, CHCs wanted to offer, in their view, an important community-based alternative for Medicaid "consumers." Finally, CHCs wanted to capitalize on their years of experience in managing Medicaid patients' care. As one CHC representative put it: "We've been doing managed care for thirty years (#26)."

Despite these reasoned arguments in favor of creating their own MCO, many other participants involved in the public discussions (either on the Council or members of the sub-committees) expressed concerns privately. First, they questioned whether a CHC-based MCO would have enough financial reserves to stay afloat if they ended up with a "bad" risk pool. Second, many found it offensive that publicly funded CHCs, with a mission to serve the indigent, would become an insurance company that competes with commercial insurers over Medicaid clients. In their view, this action contaminates CHCs' mission. Finally, as mentioned above, many were worried about the financial viability of individual clinics because by creating their own MCO, and not contracting with other MCOs, each clinic could lose some of their Medicaid clients if they sign-up with other plans.

At base, the debate hinged on whether participants thought CHCs should "empower" themselves by creating their own MCO so they could compete within the new Medicaid managed care environment. Or, whether participants thought CHCs–as publicly funded clinics– should "play along" with the MMC reforms. Privately, twenty-two percent of participants expressed a belief that CHCs should not compete with commercial plans in the MMC program, but simply "play along." Because the "collective will" of the state had decided that the use of MCOs was best for Medicaid enrollees, many participants saw CHCs' action to create their own MCO as self-interested–not in the best interest of Medicaid recipients–and subverting the will of the state.

With this as a backdrop, the fact that the CHCs in Connecticut could not agree among themselves about how to create an MCO did not bode well for their public image. In the process of creating their MCO, there was a rift among the CHCs and eventually they split and ended up creating two community-based MCOs. Thus, with two CHC-created MCOs concerns about CHCs' financial viability under the MMC reform were heightened. While concerns were heightened, many participants had mixed feelings about CHCs. They worried about CHC financial viability because the centers represent such an important source of care in poor, under-served communities. Yet, they also felt less sympathetic– some even angry–toward CHCs because they believed CHCs acted in a purely self-interested way. As publicly funded organizations serving the indigent, many participants were appalled that CHCs would act in the best interest of their organizations–and not in the best interests of the indigent. Of course, CHCs argued that acting to make their organizations as financially strong as possible was in the best interest of their clients.

With these contrasting views of CHC behavior, open public discussion about the role of CHCs in MMC reform was difficult. Prior to implementation, DSS conducted a competitive bid process to determine which plans would be given the default status–recipients who do not chose a plan are automatically assigned to default plans. As mentioned above, two commercial MCOs were awarded the default status. Perhaps not surprisingly, the two CHC-based plans (as well as a hospital-based plan) were upset that they did not win the default contract. They believed that DSS was biased in favor of commercial MCOs, and thought their experience with Medicaid patients should have given them a competitive advantage. As one CHC-plan representative put it: "We should have been given default plan status since we have been the traditional providers of care all along. If the default plan status was chosen under the criteria of access, then a commercial insurer should not have been selected (#62)." And, alluding to the fact that CHCs have been in the community taking care of the indigent for the last thirty years when no else would take them, he added: "Where were these plans when we needed them? (MMCC; December 8, 1995)"

Aside from MCO representatives, few participants publicly commented on or discussed the health plan selection process. However, many participants privately expressed concerns that the state did not set up a fair game of competition among the plans. In particular, half of the participants believed traditional Medicaid providers were treated unfavorably (or, conversely, that commercial plans received favorable treatment). Despite a real difference in opinion expressed privately, the public discussion was lopsided. For example, when a state legislator (who has long been an advocate of CHCs) asked a representative of a CHC-plan "to speak to the commercial insurers' claim that CHCs refused to contract with them," the CHC plan representative gave the following response:

> The suggestion is CHCs have done something wrong. You must understand, DSS fundamentally changed the delivery system. Now *you're blaming us* for doing something we've done for years and done well. We've developed our own MCO. We've been here for 27 years; we're a place in the community. (#62; MMC Council Meeting; December, 1995).

The state legislator responded with questions that implied she did not believe the CHC plans could compete with large commercial insurers and thought it irresponsible for them to try: "Why not contract with commercial plans? Can you withstand Department of Insurance regulation? Are you financially viable? (#6)" In his efforts to respond to these questions, no else on the Council came to CHCs' defense; despite support expressed privately.

The suggestion that CHCs were creations of their communities and therefore deserved to be independent–not beholden to commercial insurers– was never responded to when he said it publicly and never addressed again for the remainder of the eighteen months of deliberation we observed. Yet, when we asked in our private interviews "whether it is important to include traditional providers in the MMC program?," the majority (66%) said "yes" specifically *because* CHCs are community-based

organizations that have experience and expertise with the Medicaid population and an involvement and understanding of the broader community. Why wasn't this view discussed in the public forum? Why didn't
any participants (other than the one CHC representative described
above) publicly discuss the role of CHCs in underserved communities
and how this role fits with MMC reform?

Note, this issue also relates to the larger goal of improving access to
mainstream health care services. Starting back in the late 1960s, the mo-
tivation for creating CHCs in part grew out of a failure of Medicaid to
fulfill its promise of providing poor families access to mainstream
health care services. As mentioned above in relation to the topic of using School-based Health Centers (SBHCs) to improve dental access,
one response to Medicaid's mainstreaming failure was to create publicly subsidized CHCs in under-served communities. CHCs were sup-
posed to fulfill many goals. First and foremost, because many of the
poor had no primary care provider and received their care in a haphaz-
ard fashion often using emergency room settings as their primary source
of medical care, CHCs were suppose to improve access *and* the continuity of care received. It was hoped, for example, that CHCs would be able
to provide poor pregnant women with necessary pre-natal care to reduce
infant mortality rates and the problems associated with low birth weight
babies. Second, as the name implies, CHCs were suppose to reflect the
needs and desires of the *community*. Operationally, this meant the board
was composed of community representatives and–to the extent possible–staff should be hired from the surrounding community. Moreover,
the CHC would also act as an information center about services available in
the community and connect clients to other needed social service agencies.

Thus, when the CHC representative mentioned CHCs' 27-year history, he is referring to the fact that CHCs have been a presence in poor
communities specifically because the vast majority of private practicing
physicians have been unwilling to see poor patients. Yet, when these
broader issues of mainstreaming and the role of CHCs were raised, no
one responded publicly. The Council could have had a discussion about
what they hoped commercial insurers would achieve with regard to
mainstreaming, and what the role of CHCs should be given new efforts
to attract private physicians to the program. These are crucial questions
about improving access to health care for the poor, something the Connecticut legislature and the MMC Council agreed was an important goal
to obtain (or at least strive for). Unfortunately, despite various aspects
of the goal emerging in public discussion at different points in time, participants either largely ignored or severely restricted discussion about

this goal in public forums. The only topic related to this goal where prolonged discussion prevailed was the issue of creating common MCO contracting forms to alleviate the administrative burden associated with participating in MMC for dentists and other providers. Although the goal of this policy was to improve provider participation, discussion focused on incremental changes–how to maintain participation at pre-MMC levels. Thus, while conceptually related, the actual discussion about this policy seemed far removed from the larger mainstreaming goal.

ACTIVE DISCUSSION ABOUT THE TECHNICAL ASPECTS OF COST AND QUALITY

Starting with the first meeting we observed program costs were repeatedly raised in the public forum, though the discussions were never simple or straightforward. To the contrary, participants often commented about the complexity of the rate setting methodology that the state used to pay MCOs and the difficulty in understanding it. Despite the complexity, however, participants continued to raise the topic, voice concerns and ask questions. For example, after a technical presentation on the methodology behind DSS's decision to lower its average payments to MCOs from $155 to $142 a month, there was time for participants of the MMC Council ask questions and discuss the issue. State Senator Prague began with a rather detailed question and then interrupted herself saying, "oh never mind, I think the numbers will just blow my mind here." And, yet, rather than giving up she persisted with a more straightforward question: "Does each plan get $142 per member per month?" The consultant replied, "There are 48 separate rates for each plan. The debate about the $142 is about what the real average should be (February 2, 1996)." Other members of the Council then responded by asking extensive questions about the rates for newborns, whether and how DSS would compensate for MCO losses under these lower rates, and how the cost of new eligible groups–foster care children and pregnant women–would be factored into the rate. After this discussion, the provider representative for the Council concluded:

Provider rep: I'm *not* confident that rate is right.
DSS Consultant: I feel *very* confident that this rate is right.

Provider rep: We are going to expand access based on this rate, and I'm *not* convinced the plans don't have something to be concerned about.

Two Medicaid advocates then asked:

Medicaid advocate #1: "Someone suggested rates would go up, not down. MCOs were counting on an increase in the rates. Help me understand why these differences exist. Help the layperson understand.

DSS Consultant: "It is very complicated; there are so many factors. . .

Medicaid advocate #1: "Ok, I know, it's very complicated, and that it is beyond me, but help at the policy level. [For example,] how is Fairfield county $123 and Tolland county $179? What does this tell us?

DSS Consultant: "We can quantify the numbers and show that these numbers are persisting year after year. You should not infer poorer access where the rates are lower. A lot of research still cannot answer why such variations occur.

Medicaid advocate #2: "But, this *does* reflect differences in access. Do we want to pay based on regional variations that currently exist? Do we want to perpetuate those variations?"

This public exchange reveals that lay participants were not afraid to challenge technical experts even when they acknowledged a lack of full understanding about the topic. The differences in the rates between counties just did not make intuitive sense to most people on the Council or those participating in the subcommittees. Many participants kept asking: "Why is it that Fairfield County has the highest cost of living and yet is given the lowest capitation rate?" Therefore, despite a detailed explanation from technical experts, many participants remained skeptical, and pressed to figure out what they disagreed with in the technical methodology. Selected representatives, including advocates for the poor, provider representatives, and elected officials, did not defer to technical experts. Despite substantial disagreement and a publicly acknowledged lack of understanding, they pressed forward to reconcile their views with the numbers.

Similarly, they actively engaged in technical discussions about how to measure the quality of care provided by MCOs and how to measure whether recipients were getting adequate access to health and social services. As mentioned above, three of the four subcommittees emerged out of specific concerns about quality and access. Initially, discussions in these subcommittees focused on whether the MMC program was providing access to services and quality of care as the program "promised." Of course, many promises were made; thus, the subcommittees' focus could have gone in a number of directions. For example, as stated above, providing access to mainstream health care services was a stated goal under Medicaid managed care reform legislation and in the MMC Council's early documents. Thus, representatives of the poor could have held up this promise–access to mainstream medical care as a goal; and commercial plans, therefore, as the relevant comparison group to determine adequate quality for the program.

Instead, "the promise" came to be commonly understood in public discussion as "at least as good as the previous fee-for-service (FFS) Medicaid program." Privately, most participants expressed a desire that the program provide more than FFS, but they were sufficiently worried about MCOs shirking their responsibilities that many settled for "at least as good as FFS." For example, all three subcommittees focused on establishing baseline data to evaluate whether the MMC program was at least as good as FFS. The Quality Assurance (QA) subcommittee spent hours discussing various parameters to measure quality of care under the MMC program. But, never discussed what the appropriate comparison should be. The Access subcommittee devoted hours of work to developing a common credentialing form for MCOs to use for dentists so that dentists would not be burdened with eleven different forms and would perhaps be encouraged to participate in the program. Its main focus was on trying to get at least all those dentists who participated under Medicaid FFS to sign contracts with MCOs under the MMC program. Finally, the behavioral health subcommittee pursued both of these strategies–a common form for behavioral health providers and efforts to develop parameters to measure quality.

Determining how to measure quality–actually defining the parameters to use–is a particularly difficult process and took hours of committee work. At every MMC Council meeting someone from the subcommittees raised the issue of baseline data and asked what DSS was doing to measure quality and access. The conversations never amounted to much because the typical DSS response was: "yes, we will look into that," or "yes, we can incorporate that into our analysis," or "no, those data are not available." Part of the reason DSS's responses were elusive is that they just did not know yet. Although the federal government requires states to hire an external organization to monitor access and quality,

DSS was still lacking a signed contract a year after implementation began. Not surprisingly, MMC Council members were quite upset about the lack of progress and every month they would ask DSS about their efforts to develop baseline data and plans to monitor the program. When, in January of 1997, DSS hired a local organization to monitor the program, many Council members–including advocates–expressed great concern that they be involved in the process of designing a QA program. As a result, DSS agreed to meet with the subcommittees to incorporate their recommendations.

In the end, subcommittee participants did influence the process. Some of their quality parameters were included DSS's contract with the QA vendor. And, yet, for all the hours spent, it was always an incremental view of progress. Never, did they think about how they might amass data on different groups to use as a relevant comparison. The relevant comparison was always viewed as the FSS baseline, with the hope that the program would be incrementally better than before. Despite openly expressed concerns about how dismal medical quality and access to services were under the previous FFS program, this became the agreed upon standard from which to judge the program's reform.

PUBLIC TALK ABOUT TOPICS CONSIDERED WITHIN REACH

The purpose of most advisory boards, and certainly the Medicaid Managed Care Council, was to create a forum in which the views and advice of various interested groups–those most affected by Medicaid policy–could be heard. While public discussion to advise the administering agency on policy design and implementation was the simple, stated objective, this left open a number of questions about the advisory board's "ultimate" purpose. That is, was the purpose to: (1) Voice concerns about the program that the agency would then address?; (2) Collect data to investigate or uncover potential problems?; or (3) Offer policy solutions to persistent problems? While most forums involving public discussion appear to do all three–voice concern, collect data, and offer policy recommendations–several recent studies suggest that the simple voicing of concerns is rarely done without a belief that viable action steps can be taken to address such concerns (Button & Mattson, 1999; Eliasoph, 1998). We also find that assessments of what is attainable determined whether a topic received sustained discussion. If participants could see an avenue to address a particular problem, then they would view public discussion as worth their while. If not, if there was no attainable solution, then participants viewed public discussion as wasteful at best, or politically harmful at worst.

In the case of mainstream access, four interrelated factors influenced participants' assessment of whether a solution to their concerns was attainable: political feasibility; a ready solution to the problem; a lack of data to better understand the problem; and a missing common language to talk about the problem. We conjecture that any one of these factors alone would not kill public discussion, but the combination of all four significantly stymied public discussion around the goal of improving access to mainstream medical care. For example, it was not just a conservative assessment of political feasibility that contributed to participants' decision not to discuss because they viewed the climate for all quality and access improvements in Medicaid as political infeasible. Similarly, it was not just the lack of data on mainstream access that led to silence because they could have focused on collecting data as they did with the topic of improving quality. The lack of a clear solution might have been a problem, however that didn't stop participants from at least grappling with how to "solve" dental access even though many expressed private frustration with the lack of good solutions to that problem. We surmises that perhaps the most important factor for the lack of public discussion was that participants did not share a common language (or any language) to enable them to comfortably discuss mainstream access. While participants could draw on many studies about indicators of quality health care, there are few studies (actually none that we know of) that discuss measures for determining improvements in mainstream access. Many studies discuss the need to increase the number of participating physicians in the Medicaid program, but few discuss what the extent of participation should look like to break down the barriers of a two-tiered system. Perhaps this explains why the incremental claim–Medicaid managed care has expanded the number of physicians beyond Medicaid fee-for-service–was so effective at stifling public discussion. Indeed, when we asked participants whether differential treatment within Medicaid was fair? Participants reacted quite strongly to the term: "what is fairness?" "what do you mean by fair?" When we said we wanted their view of fairness, many at first felt that this was not something they could assess. After consideration, however, most came to the conclusion that differential treatment was fair if the poor were incremental better off then they were under the status quo. Thus, perhaps the reason the mainstreaming goal was so difficult to discuss in public is because most participants believe in incremental fairness.

CONCLUSION

The great promise of participatory democracy is that the state can be ruled by "the people" when they freely engage in multiple types of political action. For example, they can openly discuss their views, protest against a law they disagree with, attend town meetings to discuss a policy proposal, and safely vote for the candidate of their choice. Because an active citizenry is the central ingredient to a well functioning democracy, there is cause for concern when citizens are inactive. Just as there are many ways for citizens to be politically active in an open society, there are many ways to be inactive. Some people choose not to vote, others never contribute or join interest groups that might represent their views, others may never attend a town hall meeting, still others may participate in public meetings to discuss policies or programs that impact their lives, such as the PTO at their child's school, but choose to only voice some of their concerns.

It is this latter form of inaction–the choice to *not* raise or discuss an issue you care about–that is the focus of this chapter. However, a critique that potentially undermines the significance of this focus comes from Mackie (1998) who argues that public silence should be accepted as a legitimate expression of underlying preferences. In other words, Mackie and others (Crawford & Sobel, 1982; Ross, 1995; Elster, 1998) argue that just as individuals can misrepresent their preferences through strategically trading votes and bargaining, so to can individuals misrepresent their preferences through deliberation by what they chose to say and not say in a public forum and how they say it. Thus, one should view this form of political inaction as a legitimate form of political action, and there is no need for concern. Is restrictive public talk and incrementalism the best we can hope for from participatory democracy or, more precisely, from an intentionally inclusive advisory committees?[10]

Clearly, when able representatives chose not to raise an issue of concern in a public forum they are making a strategic decision not to speak. We argue, however, that encouraging participants to publicly discuss issues of concern has the potential to create a range of societal benefits that can be summarized into five main outcomes. First, public discussion may not change individual opinions, but may create a greater understanding, and with this, more tolerance for opposing views (Gutmann & Thompson, 1996; Walzer, 1983). Second, through the process of discussion, deliberation can encourage a public-spirited way of thinking about social problems. Through the process of exchanging ideas and beliefs, individuals may begin to think about their community, or their state or country, and not just their own self-interest (Gutmann & Thompson, 1996; Macedo, 1999). As political theorist Hanna Pitkin says about a public-spirited way of talking:

> [It] forces us to transform "I want" into "I am entitled to," a claim that becomes negotiable by public standards. In the process [of making such claims] we learn to think about the standards themselves, about our stake in the existence of standards, of justice, of our community, even of our opponents and enemies in the community; so that afterwards we are changed (1981; p. 347).[9]

Public discussion about mainstream access might transform the discussion from–how many physicians should participate in the Medicaid program?–to what type of health care facilities should the poor have access to and should that be the same as what we have access to? Are separate public clinics adequate?"

A third potential benefit may be that deliberation helps participants clarify and refine their own positions on issues. Public discourse matters a great deal for how we frame public problems and determines the range of solutions we may consider for addressing problems. How concerns are voiced, helps determine how we respond to them; and whether concerns are voiced *at all*, largely determines whether we *ever* do anything about them (Schattschneider, 1960; Gaventa, 1980; Pitkin, 1981; Eliasoph, 1998). Thus, discussion may offer new solutions, and lack of discussion may preclude certain worthy solutions, to solve social problems.[10] This is exactly the concern about the lack of public discussion about the goal of mainstream access. If participants preclude discussion about the topic then it is difficult to imagine how we will ever do anything that moves the Medicaid program, or health care for the poor more generally, away from a two-tiered system of care.

Another line of reasoning is that deliberation could lead to more just outcomes. It is widely accepted that social and economic inequality leads to political inequality because certain groups are socially and economically excluded and marginalized. As discussed in the beginning of this chapter, the poor and minority groups are significantly underrepresented in the U.S. political system. In light of existing political inequality, Iris Young, discusses how deliberative democracy could be used to widen democratic inclusion and break the cycle of political inequality by uncovering more just policies. Again, if basic discussion about the fundamental goal of a program is not discussed it is difficult to imagine how the cycle could be broken.

In considering the development of social policy in health care for the poor, we argue that participatory processes should be encouraged and implemented. But, based on our study findings, we suggest that participatory processes might want to make some topics for public discussion mandatory. For example, at a minimum, participants could be forced to return to all the agreed upon goals for the program or reform policy for sustain public discussion. This way the discussion would be forced to grapple with important and relevant, although perhaps difficult, questions rather than being swayed by immediate assessments of which topics are most attainable in the political realm.

Recognizing the importance of public discussion and disagreement does not guarantee that these benefits will emerge if participants do publicly discuss their greatest concerns. But, it is clear that none of the benefits will emerge if we never have the courage to engage in public discussion, and it is difficult to imagine how to reach a goal if we cannot first imagine how to talk about it.

NOTES

1. During the presidential race in 1992, the lack of health care security was a prominent issue. And, after Bill Clinton's election, for a moment, it appeared that national health insurance–the aspiration of liberal reformers since the 1940s–was an idea whose time finally had come. Of course, for political reasons too numerous and complex to explore here, Bill Clinton's health care reform plan failed to become law. As a result, efforts to something about the uninsured focused (as it did in the 1980s) on expanding Medicaid.

2. As noted above, this description is how Medicaid managed care should ideally work in theory. Of course, states and MCOs can lose money in a number of ways. For example, states that allow voluntary enrollment can lose money if MCOs realize favorable selection, whereas MCOs can lose money if they suffer from adverse risk selection.

3. Federal waivers at that time required the inclusion of federally qualified health centers in any type of Medicaid managed care reform.

4. She was the Litigation Director at Legal Aid Society of Hartford, Connecticut.

5. Information about the Department's public input/participation activities is summarized in a "Progress Report on Medicaid Managed Care" from Jim Gaito, Health Program Planning Manager for DSS to Lee Voghel, Principle Budget Analyst for the Legislative Office of Fiscal Analysis, December 30, 1994.

6. These provisions were contained in Public Act 94-5 passed in May 1995.

7. These were Hartford and New Haven counties.

8. For confidentiality reasons, participants in the deliberations have different identification numbers from those given in the private interview. Therefore, if the same number appears for quotes in the public deliberation and the private interview, the quotes do not represent the same person speaking, but two different people.

9. This quote was actually taken directly from Nina Eliasoph (1998, p. 16), which she used to make her point that open, political talk among common citizens is important.

10. Some argue further that because the deliberation can be a creative process–with participants brainstorming and generating new ideas–the process may be able to overcome (or at least lessen) the impact of limited knowledge on decisionmaking (Disch, 1995; Fearon, 1998; Gambetta, 1998). For example, the process of discussion may reveal that there is no compromise on the known set of policy alternatives, and therefore creates an incentive to think of new solutions. Thus, the end result is not only new solutions, but also a greater consensus over the policy decision.

REFERENCES

Beamer, G. 1999. *Creative Politics: Taxes & Public Goods in a Federal System.* Ann Arbor: University of Michigan Press.

Blendon, R. J., J. T. Young and C. M. DesRoches. 1999. "The uninsured, the working uninsured, and the public." *Health Affairs* 18(6): 203-211.

Button, M., and K. Mattson. 1999. "Deliberative Democracy in Practice: Challenges and Prospects for Civic Deliberation within a Representative System." *Polity* XXXI(4): 609-38.

Colburn, Don. 1991. "Pregnant Women on Medicaid Get Less Care than Others." *Washington Post* 29 October, Z5.

Congressional Research Service (CRS). 1993. *Medicaid Source Book: Background Data and Analysis (A 1993 Update).* Washington, D.C.: U.S. Government Printing Office.

Connecticut General Assembly, Office of Fiscal Analysis. 1994. *Fiscal Year 1995 Budget Projections.*

Coughlin, T. A., L. Ku, and J. Holahan. 1994. *Medicaid since 1980: Costs, Coverage, and the Shifting Alliance between the Federal Government and the States.* Washington, DC: The Urban Institute.

Crawford, V. P., and J. Sobel. 1982. "Strategic Information Transmission." *Econometrica* 50(6): 1431-51.

Dalleck, Geraldine. 1996. "A Consumer Advocate on Medicaid Managed Care." *Health Affairs* 15(3): 174-177.

Davidson, Stephen M. and Stephen A. Somers. 1998. *Remaking Medicaid: Managed Care for the Public Good.* San Francisco: Jossey-Bass Inc., Publishers.

Eliasoph, N. 1999. *Avoiding Politics: How Americans Produce Apathy in Everyday Life.* New York: Cambridge University Press

Elster, J. 1998. "Introduction." In *Deliberative Democracy*, ed., J. Elster, 1-18. New York: Cambridge University Press.

Friedman, Thomas L. 1993. President Allows States Flexibility on Medicaid Funds. *New York Times*, 2 February, A1.

Gaventa. J. 1980. *Power and Powerlessness: Quiescence and Rebellion in an Appalachian Valley* Illinois: University of Illinois Press and Oxford: Clarendon Press.

Gold, M. 1996. "Medicaid managed care: Lessons from five states." *Health Affairs* 15(3): 153-166.

Grogan, C. M. 1997. "The Medicaid managed care policy consensus for welfare recipients: A reflection of traditional welfare concerns" *Journal of Health Politics, Policy and Law* 22(3): 815-838.

Grogan, C. M., and M. K. Gusmano. 2005. "State-Level Deliberative Democracy: A Case Study of Deliberation in Practice." *State Politics & Policy Quarterly* 5(2): 126-146.

Grogan, C. M., and M. K. Gusmano. 1999. "How are safety-net providers faring under Medicaid managed care?" *Health Affairs* 18(2): 233-237.

Gutmann, A., and D. Thompson. 1996. *Democracy and Disagreement.* Cambridge, MA: MIT Press.

Gutmann, A., and D. Thompson. 1999. Democratic Disagreement. In *Deliberative Politics: Essays on Democracy and Disagreement*, ed., S. Macedo, 243-80. Oxford University Press.

Habermas, J. 1984. *The Theory of Communicative Action, I and II.* Boston: Beacon Press.

Habermas, Jurgen, 1990. *Moral Consciousness and Communicative Ethics.* (Cambridge, MA: MIT Press)

Holahan, J., S. Zuckerman, A. Evans, and S. Rangarajan. 1998(b). "Medicaid Managed Care in Thirteen States." *Health Affairs* 17(3): 43-63.

Horvath, I., and N. Kaye: 1995. *Medicaid Managed Care: A Guide for States, First Edition.* Portland, ME: National Academy for State Health Policy.

Hurley, R. E., and S. A. Somers. 2003. "Medicaid and managed care: A lasting relationship?" *Health Affairs* 22(1): 77-88.

Iglehart, J. K. 1999. "The American Health Care System: Medicaid" *NEJM* 340(5): 403-408.

Macedo, S. 1999. Introduction. In *Deliberative Politics: Essays on Democracy and Disagreement*, ed., S. Macedo, 3-16. New York: Oxford University Press.

Mackie, G. 1998. "All Men Are Liars: Is Democracy Meaningless?" In *Deliberative Democracy*, ed., J. Elster, 69-96. Cambridge: Cambridge University Press.

Mansbridge, Jane. 1980. *Beyond Adversary Democracy.* N.Y.: Basic Books.

Oliver, T. R. 1998. "The collision of economics and politics in Medicaid managed care: Reflections on the course of reform in Maryland." *Milbank Quarterly* 76(1): 59-102.

Pitkin, H. 1981. *The Concept of Representation.* Berkeley: University of California Press.

Rowland, Diane, Judith Feder and Alina Salganicoff. 1993. "Research reports–Medicaid Financing Crisis: Balancing Responsibilities, Priorities, and Dollars." *The Wilson Quarterly* 17(4): 136

Ross, L. 1995. "Reactive Devaluation in Negotiation and Conflict Resolution." In *Barriers to Conflict Resolution*, eds., K. Arrow et al., 26-43. New York: Norton.

Schattschneider, E. E. 1960. *The Semisovereign People: A Realist's View of Democracy in America.* Hinsdale, Illinois: The Dryden Press.

Slovut, Gordon. 1991. Many Kids under 5 Lack Shots, HMO Says. *Star Tribune* (Minneapolis, Minnesota), 28 June, 3B.

Sunstein, C. R. 1998. Health-Health Trade-offs. In *Deliberative Democracy*, ed., J. Elster, 232-59. Cambridge University Press.

U.S. Senate, Committee on Finance. 1967. Social Security Amendments of 1967, Part 3. 90th Cong., 1st sess., 20-22 and 26 September.

Williams, L. 1994. "State Lags in Setting Up Cost Controls for Medicaid." *Hartford Courant* December 16: A1.

Young, I. M. 2000. *Inclusion and Democracy*. Oxford, UK: Oxford University Press.

INDEX

AARP 47, 48, 49
abortion
  campaigns against clinics 108,
    112, 114, 118
  legalization of 107
  rights 106, 117
    curtailment of 113, 118-19
  services 105
access to services 92, 140, 147
  measuring 142-3, 144
  and Medicaid managed care 123,
    125, 126
  for women 105-6
ACE (Acute Care of the Elderly)
    units 36
  in hospitals 36-7
activities of daily living (ADL) 27
  and ACE units 36
  informal caregiving 48, 49
  PACE 4
Adams, D. 69, 72
advanced illness care 26, 27
advocacy
  for family caregivers 57, 58-9,
    61, 62
    on-line support 59
  feminist groups 106
  for poor 131
  Womancare 117
Aging, Administration on 53
aging population 47, 60, 97
Alary, J. 94
Albert, S.M. 49
Alberta: regional devolution 75, 76
Aliotta, S. 15
Alzheimer's Association 58-9
ambulatory care: Quebec 96, 97
anti-abortion campaigns 108, 112,
    114, 118

Archambault, C. 77
Armey, R. 113
Arno, P.S. 60, 61
Atherly, A.J. 6
Austin, B. 26

Bader, E. 113, 118, 119
Badgley, F.R. 74
Baird, K. 109
Baird-Windle, P. 113, 118, 119
Bajorska, A.M. 6, 42
Balanced Budget Act (1997) 7, 28,
    37-8
Banting, K.G. 71
Beamer, G. 124
Béland, F. 38, 77
Bélanger, J.P. 90
Bengtson, V.L. 47
Bennett-Haigney, L. 108, 118
Bergman, H. 38
Bershadsky, B. 13, 37, 40, 41
Besdine, R.W 26
Bhatia, V. 75
Bird, R.M. 69, 73
black people
    caregivers' hours 48
    survival advantage under PACE 6
Black Women's Health Project 107
Blancato, R.B. 52
Blendon, R.J. 124
Bloom, B.S. 37
Boase, J.P. 69
Bodenheimer, T. 3, 9, 10
Boivin, R. 87
Bonin, L. 77
Boston Women's Health Book
    Collective 106-7, 109
Boudreau, A. 76
Boult, C. 15, 35

Bourque, D. 93
Branch, L.G. 6, 7
Brizius, J.A. 60
Brown, D.M. 71
Brown, L.D. 67
Brown, R. 15
Brzuzy, S. 119
Burstein, N. 6
Bush administration and women's
    healthcare 107-8, 118-19
Button, M. 144

Cafferata, G.L. 47, 48
Cameron, D. 68, 69
Campos, P. 108
Canada 67-81
    Health and Social Transfer grant
        71, 72-3
    mental health statistics 97
    see also fiscal federalism
Canada Health Act (1984) 67, 71
    compliance 70
    and federalism 68-70
    provisions of 68
capitation funding 32, 37, 39, 42
Cardwell, M. 77
caregiver organizations 1, 56-61, 62
    challenges to policy-making 56-8
caregiving 48-9
    hours provided 48
    private-public dichotomy 49-50
    see also family
Carlson, B. 54
Caro, F.G. 61
Carpenter, L. 55-6
case management and CMS 30-1
    functions of 31
Cash and Counseling services 54-5, 61
Cassel, C.K. 26
CEI (Center for Elders Independence)
    3, 11
CGA (Comprehensive Geriatric
    Assessment) 35
Chadiha, L.A. 59
Champoux, L. 91
Charles, C.A. 74
Chatterji, P. 6, 14
Chen, A. 15
Chen, Q. 6
Chodos, H. 77
Christian Conservatives 107

Chronic Care Consortium, National 12
chronic care/illness 3
    consumer empowerment 19-20
    and group visit models 34-5
    Medicare Advantage 15-16
    see also PACE
Clair Commission 77, 78
Clark, L. 108
Clark, M.L. 6
Clarkson, F. 118
Clinton, President Bill 124
CLSCs (Centres Locaux des Services
    Communautaires) 2, 77, 78, 87-100
    1980s mandate 92-3
    2004-5 reforms 98-9
    community action 88, 90, 91, 93,
        94, 96, 98, 99
    and community organizations 95-6
    community organizers 88, 89, 93-5
    creation of 89-91, 99-100
    development of culture 94
    financing 90
    implementation of 90-1
    inequalities in development 92
    and local service networks 98-9
    mental health services 97-8
    merger with hospital centers 89
    three models 88, 91, 96, 99
CMS (Centers for Medicare and
    Medicaid Services) 27-33
    building research capacity 29
    case management 30-1
    children's health insurance 28
    consumer choice 30
    financial incentives 31-3
    improving health of population 29
    improving quality of care 29
    monitoring and evaluating 28
    population health and
        expenditures 33
    prescription drugs 29
    research and evaluation program
        27, 28-9, 42
        current themes 28-9
    vulnerable populations 27, 30
    within levels of care 30
Coalition for the Medical Rights for
    Women 107
Colburn, D. 124
Coleman, B. 13, 52
Coleman, E.A. 12, 35

Coleman, N. 55
collective action, feminist health
  care 109
Collin, J.P. 87
community action 88, 90, 91, 93, 94,
  96, 98, 99
Community Health Centers (CHCs)
    Connecticut 133, 136-41
    creation of own MCOs 137-8, 139
    enabling services 137
    Quebec 89
community organizations 95-6
community organizers 88, 89, 93-5
    professionalization 95
comprehensive medicine 88
condition management 26, 27
Connecticut 123, 126-45
    DSS 'diplomacy campaign' 128, 129
    Medicaid costs 126
    Medicaid managed care 2, 123,
    126-9
        Council 129
        enrollment rates 129-30
consumer choice
    Cash and Counseling services 54-5
    and CMS 30, 42, 44
consumer empowerment 19-20
continuity of care 14
continuum of care 25-7, 42, 44
    compartmentalization of 25
    three dimensions of 26
contraception rights 105, 106, 107
    curtailment of 113
Contract with America 113
cooperative federalism 68, 71
Cordon, S. 71
Coughlin, T.A. 124
Coulam, R.F. 6
Courchene, T.J. 68, 71
Covinsky, K.E. 6, 36, 42
Crawford, V.P. 146
CSSS (Centre de Santé et des
  Services Sociaux) 2, 79
Curbow, B. 109

Dailard, C. 108
Dalleck, G. 126, 133
D'Amour, D. 94
Davidson, S.M. 124
day centers, adult 5, 12
    attendance and PACE 8, 9, 38, 40

Deber, R.B. 74
Defense of Marriage Act (1996) 113
dental care 131-6, 140, 145
    access to mainstream dentists
    132-5
    dental hygienists 134-5
    practitioner participation 131-2,
    133, 141
    public funded clinics 133
DesRoches, C.M. 124
DHHS (Department of Health and Human
  Services) 33
Dickinson, H. 75
disabled people 28
    PACE 5-6
    women 107
discharge from hospital
    discharge planners 31
    and family caregivers 49-50
disease management 34-6, 42-3
Dixon-Miller, R. 105
Dobell, L. G. 25-44
domestic violence 105
Dorsey, T. 7
Downer, Carol 106
Driver, D. 75
Dyck, B. 118

Eddy, L. 57
Ehrenreich, B. 17, 106
Ehrenreich, J. 17
Eleazer, G.P. 4
Eleazer, P. 38
Eliasoph, N. 144, 147
Elster, J. 146
empowerment, consumer 6, 19-20
    feminist health care 109
Eng, C. 4, 5, 6, 7, 10, 20, 38, 39,
  42
England, S.E. 50
English, D. 106
Equalization Program 71, 72-4
Established Programs Financing Act
  69-70
    EFP arrangement 70-1
Estes, C.L. 3-20, 60, 61
Estes, S.B. 51
EverCare 19, 32, 37, 41

Families USA Foundation 126
Family Caregiver Alliance 59

family caregivers
  demands on 49
  devaluing of 57-8
  financial penalties 60
  and FMLA 51-2
  funding for support programs 52, 53
  hours per week 48
  importance of 47
  legislative support 51-6
  Medicaid Waiver Programs 53-6
  and NFCSP 52-3, 57, 58, 61-2
  numbers of 47
  policies 50-6, 60
    difficulties 56-8
  post-hospital discharge 49-50
  and social security benefits 60-1
  strategies for policy advocacy 58-9
  work-home demands 49
  see also caregiver organizations
family involvement in PACE 5
Family and Medical Leave Act 51-2, 57, 58
  limitations of 52, 61-2
family medicine groups 88
Favreau, L. 95, 96
Feder, J. 124
federalism and Canada Health Act 68-70
  see also fiscal federalism
Feinberg, L.F. 47, 52, 53, 54, 61
Feldt, G. 113, 118, 119
feminist health care 105-20
  see also Womancare
feminist health movement 108-9
  and self-help 105
Feminist Majority Fund 108
Feminist Women's Health Center 113
Fierlbeck, K. 69
Finance Canada 70, 71, 72-3, 74
financial aspects of PACE 4, 5, 7, 16, 37
financial incentives, CMS 31-3
fiscal federalism 1, 68, 81
  current issues 73-4
  equalization issues 73-4
  level of federal contribution 73
  significance of 70-3
  and tax points 73
Fitzgerald, P. 8
Flanders, D. 13

Flanders, L. 118
Fleury, M.-J. 79, 87-101
Flood, S. 37, 41
Florida 13
Fooks, C. 74
Foote, S.M. 26, 34
for-profit providers and PACE 9-10, 19
Forest, P.-G. 67-81
Foster, L. 54
Foster, S.E. 60
Fox, N. 4, 38
Fox, P.D. 15
FoxGrage, W. 52
fragmentation of care and group programs 35
Friedman, T.L. 125

Gaumer, B. 87-101
Gaventa, J. 147
Geary, M.A. 105, 107, 109
Gelb, J. 105, 107, 108, 109
GEM (geriatric evaluation and management) programs 34, 35-6
gender inequities 105
geriatric care 34, 35-6
  see also PACE
Giarusson, R. 47
Gillespie, E. 113
Gingrich, N. 113
Glass, J.L. 51
Godbout, J. 87
Gold, M. 126
Goldberg, S.C. 18
Goldensen, S.M. 18
Gottleib, L. 77
Grey, G. 69, 75
Grogan, C.M. 123-49
Gross, D.L. 4, 5, 7-8, 9, 10, 40
Grothaus, L.C. 12, 35
group visit models 34-5
Gusmano, M.K. 123-49
Gutmann, A. 146, 147

Hansen, Jenny Chin 8
Hardy, B. 57
Harrington, M. 60
Hart, A. 49
Hawley-McDonald, G. 78
Haynes, K.S. 58, 59
health care service delivery, Canada 67-81

2004 funding agreement 71-2
basic insured services 68
equalization payments 69, 71, 72-4
federal funding amounts 69-70
federal/provincial relationship
68-9
hospital costs 75
health care system: gender
inequities 105
health condition prevention 26
health cooperatives 106
health plans and Medicaid 136-41
health promotion: CLSCs 89
Heisler, M.O. 67, 68, 80
Helfgot, J. 118
Heller, K. 117
Herd, P. 50
Hernandez, M. 3-20
Heuglin, T.O. 68, 69
Hill, S. 105, 109
HIV/AIDS services 105, 109
Womancare 116
curtailment 113
HMOs
and family caregivers 56
and PACE 16
Holahan, J. 124, 125-6, 133
Holtzman, J. 6
Home and Community Based Services 54,
55-6
home support programs: Quebec 97
Homeless Women's Health Outreach
Project 116
Homyak, P. 13, 40, 41
Horvath, I. 125
Hospice and Advanced Illness
Coordinated Care programs 29
hospice care 32
hospitalization rates
and CGA 35
effect of PACE 6, 39
and MSHO 41
hospitals
Canadian expenditure 75
discharge 'quicker and sicker'
49-50
Howell-White, S. 15
HRSA (Health Resources and Services
Administration) 33
Hurley, J. 75
Hurley, R.E. 125

Hurtubise, Y. 95, 96
Hyde, C.A. 105-20

IADL tasks 27
informal caregiving 48, 49
iatrogenic complications, preventing
36
ideology and health care 17
Iglehart, J.K. 125, 126
Illston, L.H. 7, 9
Immergut, E. 74
inequalities
gender 105
social and economic 147
informal caregiving services 48
see also family caregivers
information systems, PACE 5
institutional care as policy focus
50, 54
insurance
children's health 28
health plans and Medicaid 136-41
and PACE 16-17
social 18, 19
integrated care 13, 25-44
ACE units 36
difficulties with 14
disease management 34-6
experience with 33-42
inpatient integration
interventions 36-7
PACE 1-10
state programs 13-15
Internet and caregivers' support 59
Irvin, C.V. 7

Jackman, J. 108
Jayadevappa, R. 37
Jha, A.K. 6
Johnson, R.W. 51, 53
Johri, M. 38

Kaiser Foundation 89
Kane, R.A. 13, 48
Kane, R.L. 6, 7, 9, 13, 37, 40, 41,
42, 48
Karon, S.L. 39
Katz, R. 26
Kaufman, T. 77
Kaye, N. 125
Keckhafer, G. 37

Keigher, S.M. 50, 54
Khoury, A. 109
Kidder, D. 6
Koenig, E. 108
Kolk, A. 108
Kouri, D. 75
Kraynak, M.A. 105, 109
Kronenfeld, J. 119
Ku, L. 124
Kunitz, S. 4, 5, 40
Kushner, C. 78

Lachapelle, R. 95
Ladd, R.C. 13
Laghi, B. 72
Lavizzo-Mourey, R. 37
Leader, J. 108
Lechner, V.M. 52
Lee, J.A. 15
Lee, M. 42
lesbian health care 107, 108, 109, 116
Leseman, F. 94
Levine, C. 49, 60, 61
life expectancy, US 47
Linsk, N.L. 50
Lomas, J. 74, 75, 76
long term care
    CMS program 27
    PACE as model 12-15
    policy focus 50
    political economy issues 17-19
    pressure for reform 18
    private insurance 16-17
    US corporate interests 17, 18
    see also PACE
Lonsway, K. 108, 118
Los Angeles Feminist Women's Health Center 106
Lucas, J.A. 15
Lui, L.Y. 6, 42
Lum, Y.S. 13, 40, 41
Lundy, M. 109
Lynch, M. 3-20, 60, 61

McCann, R. 4, 38
Macedo, S. 147
McGovern, P. 49
Mackie, G. 146
Magner, G. 119
Maino, F. 71

Maioni, A. 71, 77
Managed Care Organizations (MCOs) 2, 124, 127
    accountability 133
    measuring quality 142-4
    payment rate setting 141-2
Manitoba regionalization 76-7
    Regional Health Authorities 76
market ideology 17
marketing, PACE 10
Marse, H. 67
Maruska, D. 13
MAS (Quebec Department of Social Affairs) 90, 92, 95
Maslove, A.W. 68, 71
Mason, S. 109
Massachusetts: Medicare waivers 12, 13
Massey, S. 7
Master, R.J. 4, 10, 20
Matter, D. 49
Mattson, K. 144
Medicaid managed care (MMC) 123-6
    advisory board 144
    and commercial providers 125-6
    goals of 123
    and growth of delivery networks 128
    health plan participation 136-41
    improving quality 123
    increasing access 123
    introduction of 124-5, 127-9
    objectives 128
    provider-to-patient ratios 133, 134
    public discussion topics 144-5, 146
    reducing costs 123
    two-tiered system 131
Medicaid program 2, 27
    1990s failures 123-4
    costs 126
    cuts in spending 57
    and PACE provision 5, 6, 20
Medicaid Waiver Programs 13, 14, 53-6, 61
    limitations 62
medical model 88
medical records, electronic 5
Medicare Modernization Act 15, 18, 28, 29

Medicare program 27
   Centers for Excellence
      Demonstrations 28
   Current Beneficiary Survey 33
   drug card 29
   Medicare Advantage 12, 15-16
   and PACE 5, 6, 7, 20
   privatization forces 18, 19
   waivers 12, 13, 14, 41
Memmott, M.M. 60, 61
mental health services
   female 105
   practitioner participation 132
   Quebec 97-8
MEPS (Medical Expenditures Panel
   Survey) 33
Meyer M.H. 50
Mickelson, J.S. 58, 59
Miller, E.A. 53
Miller, N.A. 7, 9
Minnesota
   Disability Health Options (MnDHO)
      12-13, 39
   HCBS program 55-6
   Medicare waivers 12, 41
   Senior Health Options (MSHO)
      12, 13, 39, 40-2
Mollica, R. 13, 14
Montgomery, A. 54, 61
Montreal: citizens' groups 87
Moore, R.J. 15
Morgan, A. 8
Morgen, S. 105, 106, 107, 108, 109,
   113, 119
Morgenbesser, M. 117
Morin, P. 77
Morris, T. 8
mortality rates: effect of PACE 6
MSSS 92, 97-8
Mukamel, D.B. 4, 6, 7, 39, 40, 42
multidisciplinary teams
   and CMS 30, 31
   PACE 4-5, 15, 38

NASUA (National Association of State
   Units on Aging) 52-3
National Alliance of Caregivers
   (NAC) 47, 48, 49, 58
National Family Caregiver Support
   Program 52-3, 57, 58
   limitations 61-2

National PACE Association 4, 16
Neal, M.B. 52
Neighbourhood Health Centers 89
New Right actions
   Womancare Health Center 110-14,
      118-19
      harassment and violence
         112-13, 114, 118
   and women's health care 107-8
Newcomer, R.J. 25-44
Newman, S. 52, 53, 61
Nichols F.H. 105, 106, 107
NLTCS (National Long Term Care
   Survey) 33
non-profit providers and PACE 9, 18
NOW (National Organization for
   Women) 107, 108, 119
nursing homes 28
   expenditure on 50
   Medicare certification 14
   and MSHO 41
   utilization 16
      effect of PACE 6, 39

O'Connor, D.L. 57, 59
O'Keeffe, J. 55-6
Older Americans Act 53
older people: growth in numbers 47,
   60, 97
Older Women's League 61
Oliver, T.R. 126, 133
Olmstead v. L.C. 55
On Lok 3, 8, 12
Ontario: regionalization 75-6, 80
Operation Rescue 108, 110, 112
Oregon 13
O'Reilly, P. 69, 71

Pacala, J.T. 6
PACE (Program for All-Inclusive Care
   for the Elderly) 1, 3-20, 25, 28,
   32, 37-42
   access for middle-income seniors 10
   barriers to growth 7-10
   broader policy implications 11-20
   care data 33
   and continuum of care 42-3
   criticisms 6-7
   and disabilities 5-6
   effectiveness 6, 20
   evaluations 39-42

family involvement 5
financial aspects 4, 5, 7, 16, 37
for-profit providers risk 9
and individual preferences 19-20
innovations fostered by 20
lack of start-up capital 9
marketing need 10
Medicaid capitation payments 37, 39
as model for state care programs 12-15, 43
number of participants and sites 7-8
and nursing home care 16
outcomes 6-7
participant characteristics 4, 37
participant empowerment 6, 19, 43
prepaid financing 4
and private insurance 16-17
privatization pressures 18-19
program characteristics 4-6
resource allocation 38
state to state variations 7
types of intervention 5
unattractiveness to some elders 8-9
Palley, E. 47-62
Palley, H.A. 67-81, 109
Palley, M.L. 105, 107, 108, 109
palliative care 26, 27
Parker, P. 13
Parrott, S. 57
Parrott, T.M. 49, 50, 58
participatory democracy 146-8
Partnership for Caring (2001) 58, 60
Paulus, A 67
Pedulla, J. 4, 38
Pemberton, D. 5
personal care: informal services 48
Peters, G.B. 67, 68, 80
Philips, B. 54, 55, 108
physicians 88, 94
    access to mainstream 129, 130
    participation in Medicaid 127, 130-1, 133-4, 136
    participation in MMC 136, 140, 145
Pitkin, H. 147
Plain, R.H.M. 74
PMAP (Prepaid Medical Assistance Program) 41
Point of Service (POS) plans 28

policies for caregiving
    lack of interest groups 57
    and public perception 57-8, 61
    role of federal government 57
    and US political system 56-7
political economy issues 17-19
political inequality 147
poor families
    and Medicaid in 1990s 124
    and Medicaid managed care 126
    women's health needs 109
population health and expenditures 33
Poupart, R. 94
Pratt, C. 57
Preferred Provider Organizations (PPOs) 28
prescription drugs 29
Price, R. 117
primary care 88, 93
    and DM interventions 36
    and inpatient care 37
PRISMA Program 7, 77
private long term care insurance 16-17
private provision and Medicaid managed care 124
private-public dichotomy 49-50
privatization of social insurance 18, 19
Prospective Payment System 49
provider-to-patient ratios 133, 134
public clinics 136
public discussion 144-5, 146-8
public-private partnerships 100

quality of care, measuring 142-4
Quebec 69
    ambulatory care 96, 97
    CLSCs 87-100
    community organizations 95-6
    health care reform 77-9, 87-9
        1970s reform 90
        1990s reform 93
        2004-5 reform 98-9
    local networks 78-9
    MAS 90, 92, 95
    MSSS 88
    Quiet Revolution 87
    Regional Health Boards 77-8
    regionalization 77-9, 80
    see also CLSCs

Rachlis, M. 78
Rasmussen, K. 68
Rassen, A. 15
Rassen, J. 15
Ratcliff, K. 109
Raziano, D.B. 37
Redden, C.J. 75
reform of health care 126-44
    Canada 74-9
      Quebec 77-9, 90, 93, 98-9
    see also Medicaid managed care
regionalization of Canadian health
   care 1, 67
    and accountability 74
    and management functions 74-5
    pressure for 74
    resources issues 76
    results 80
    shift to community-based 74, 75,
      76, 79-80
Reinharz, S. 117
reproductive choice 105
reproductive health: curtailment of
   services 118-19
Reproductive Rights National
   Network 107
    principles 106
Reuben, D.B. 26, 35, 36, 37
reverse mortgages 32
Riger, S. 117
Riley, T. 13, 14
Robinson, J. 39
Robison, S. 15
Rodriguez, C. 90
Roe v. Wade 107, 113
Rosato, N.S. 15
Ross, L. 146
Rosser, S. 105, 109
Rowland, D. 124
Rozario, P.A. 47-62
rural areas and PACE provision 8
Ruzek, S.B. 105, 106, 107, 109, 113,
   119
Ryan, J. 13, 19, 39, 40
Ryan, S.D. 42

Said Siadaty, M. 41
Salganicoff, A. 124
Sandhu, N. 12
Sangl, J. 47, 48
Sardell, A. 87

Saskatchewan: regionalization 75, 80
Sasso, A.T.L. 51, 53
Schattschneider, E.E. 147
Scheidler, J. 108, 114
Schellhas, B. 113
Schneider, B. 55
School Based Health Centers 135,
   140
Schore, J. 54
Segal, E. 119
self-help and feminist health
   movement 105
    Womancare 105, 109, 110, 111,
      115-16, 117
Senior Care Organizations (SCOs) 13
sexually transmitted diseases 109
    treatment 116
Shannon, K. 5
Sherman, A. 57
Sherwin, S. 109
SHMOs 15, 32
Siadaty, M.S. 13
Siegel, L.C. 26
Silverstein, M. 47, 49, 50, 58
Simeon, R. 68, 69
Simon-Rusinowitz, L. 50
Simpson, J. 69
Slovut, G. 124
Smith, G. 55-6
Smith, M.A. 7
Sobel, J. 146
social model 88
social policy 44
Social Security Act 54
Social Union Framework Agreement 69
Soderstrom, L. 77
Somers, S.A. 124, 125
Sparer, M. 57
Special Needs Plans (SNP) 15-16
Spurgeon, D. 70, 72
state-sponsored programs 12-15
Stevenson, D.G. 12, 14, 26
Stone, R.I. 13, 26, 47, 48, 54
storytelling for awareness raising 59
Super, N. 13, 19, 39, 40
Swan, B. 74
Swenden, W. 69
symptom management 27
Szutsu, P. 5

Tan, E.J. 6

targets, Canadian
  equalization funds 72
  waiting times 72, 73
Temkin-Greener, H. 4, 6, 7, 39, 40, 42
Texas
  Medicaid waiver programs 56
  Texas Star Plus 13
Thomas, L. 5
Thompson, D. 146, 147
Thornton, M.C. 48
Tilly, J. 54
Tousignant, P. 77
transitions between levels of care 30, 31, 33
Tronto, J. 58
Tuuk, M. 42

university hospital center: Quebec 89

Van Reenen, C. 5
Veenstra, G. 74
Villagra, V.G. 26
Vladeck, B.C. 60
vulnerable populations and CMS 27, 30, 42

Wagner, E.H. 12, 26, 35
waiting times targets: Canada 72, 73
Walker, A. 47, 57
Walter, L.C. 42
Walzer, 146
Wandersman, A. 117
Wang, H. 47
Warden, G.L. 26
Warren, D. 118
Weiner, A. 41
Weiner, J.M. 54
Weingarten, S.R. 34
Weinstein, M. 108
Weisman, C. 105, 106, 107, 108, 109
welfare state: two tier US system 18
Wessen, A.F. 68
White, A. 6
White, G. 68
White-Means, S.I. 48
Whitelaw, N.A. 26
Wieland, D. 6, 15, 39

Wiener, J.M. 12, 14, 18, 26
Williams, J.I. 75
Williams, L. 127
Wilson, J.Q. 57
Wisconsin
  DHFS 40
  Medicare waivers 12
Wisconsin Partnership Program 13, 39-40
  reported outcomes 40
Wisensale, S. 51, 52
Withorn, A. 117
Womancare Health Center 105, 109-20
  collectivist approach 115-16
  expansion of services 116, 117, 120
  founding period 110-11
  intimidation and harassment 112-13, 114
  New Right actions 110-14, 118-19
  responses to 114-17, 119, 120
  risk assessment 113
  philosophy 110
  and social change 111
  survival of 117-18

women caregivers 47
  legislative protection 51
women's health care 2
  erosion of 119
  funding reductions 108, 111-12
  initiatives 106-7
  see also Womancare
Women's Health Network, National 107
Wood, J.E. 99
Woods, J. 74
Wooldridge, J. 15
workforce, direct care 28
workplace health and safety 105
World Health Organization 88, 92

Young, I.M. 147
Young, J.T. 124

Zhang, H. 41
Zimmerman, M. 105, 109
Zimmerman, Y.A. 5, 6